W9-CTY-695

Arisal of the Clear

Arisal Of The Clear

A Simple Guide To Healthy Eating According To Traditional Chinese Medicine

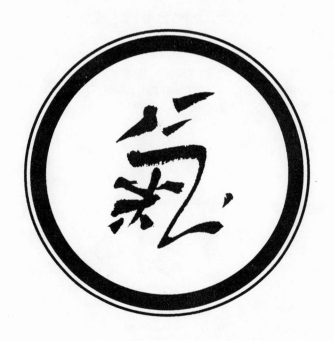

Bob Flaws

Published by:

BLUE POPPY PRESS
1775 LINDEN AVE.
BOULDER, CO 80304

FIRST EDITION
OCTOBER 1991

ISBN 0-936185-27-9
Library of Congress Catalog # 91-073954

Printed at Westview Press, Boulder, CO

This book is printed on archive quality, acid free, recycled paper.

Preface

T en years ago or more, my wife and I wrote a book on Chinese dietary therapy entitled *Prince Wen Hui's Cook*. That book, which is still in print, was meant primarily as a practitioner's guide to Chinese dietary therapy. It discussed Chinese dietary therapy in terms of TCM *bian zheng lun zhi* methodology or erecting a treatment plan based on a pattern discrimination diagnosis. Doing such a diagnosis requires considerable education and training. It is something a layperson cannot and should not do for themselves. It is a professional endeavor to do correctly. However, over the years, many patients and laypersons have attempted to use *Prince Wen Hui's Cook* as a guide to healthy eating. When those patients have returned to me with questions generated by reading *Prince*, it became clear that the information that book contains is too confusing and technically complex for their purposes. On the other hand, diet is one of the four basic foundations of good health, and, unless one eats wisely, it is difficult, if not impossible, to maintain long term good health and reap lasting results from other such therapies as Chinese herbal medicine and acupuncture.

Therefore I have decided to publish this smaller, more concise book on Chinese dietary therapy written especially for the lay reader. It is a distillation of what I continually tell my patients day in and day out. I have kept technical information regarding individual foods to a minimum and have emphasized the use of simple metaphors and similes to convey this information in an easily apprehendable way. Healthy eating is not all that complex or difficult to understand, and most people do not need extremely unique and unusual diets. The basic insights of traditional Chinese dietary therapy are relatively simple and universally applicable.

I believe that Chinese dietary theory makes the most sense of any approach to healthy eating currently available. It explains digestion and nutrition in a very immediate, common sense, and human way. It also substantiates and helps make sense of many of the latest scientific opinions about food and diet. Hopefully, this book will fill the clear and present need for a concise layperson's guide to Chinese dietary therapy. If it does, then *bon appetit* and *wan sui*, good eating and may you live ten thousand years.

Bob Flaws
Boulder, CO
July 1991

Table Of Contents

The Basics of Good Health

I n the Tang Dynasty, the famous doctor Sun Si-miao said that, when a person is sick, the doctor should first regulate the patient's diet and lifestyle. In most cases, these changes alone are enough to effect a cure over time. Sun Si-miao said that only if changes in diet and lifestyle are not enough should the doctor administer other interventions such as internal medicine and acupuncture. Although most patients coming for professional TCM treatment today do need internal medicine and/or acupuncture as well as changes in their diet and lifestyle, it is most definitely my experience that without appropriate changes in diet and lifestyle, herbs and acupuncture do not achieve their full and lasting effect.

Form & Function

There are four basic foundations of achieving and maintaining good health. These are diet, exercise, adequate rest and relaxation, and a good mental attitude. Chinese medical theory is based on yin and yang. In terms of medicine, yin means substance and yang means function. This is similar to the Western medical dichotomy between form and function. Form and function are interdependent. Substance or form is both the material, anatomical basis of function and its fuel. Function, on the other hand, activates and motivates form and also repairs, builds, and maintains it.

We can liken the human organism to a candle. A candle's function is to burn and, therefore, shed light. The flame of the candle is dependent upon its form. At the same time, the candle's form, its wick and wax, is the fuel for the candle's function. The human organism is very similar to a candle in that our various activities and consciousness are dependent upon our form, our anatomy. Our functional activities are a product of consuming and transforming or metabolizing substance. When we are young, we generate more substance than we consume and thus we are able to grow, repair, and keep our bodies youthful in shape and appearance. However, past a certain age, due to a decline in our bodily organs' efficiency, we no longer produce an excess of fuel or substance and so we begin to consume our own form. When we have consumed all our yin substance, our organism no longer has sufficient fuel for function and so ceases or dies.

Unlike the candle which is endowed with a finite, unreplenishable form at the moment of its making, we humans are capable of taking in new form or substance. We do this by breathing, eating, and drinking. It is eating and drinking which provide us with the substance which fuels our day to day activities and which is transformed into our body's material basis. Therefore, from the point of view of form or yin substance, we most definitely are what we eat, drink, and breathe.

Exercise is a type of function. It is activity. In relationship to diet, exercise is yang to diet's yin. Exercise keeps function functioning at peak efficiency. However, in Chinese medicine, exercise and rest/relaxation are seen as the yin/yang aspects of a single issue. If we are too active, *i.e.*, hyperfunctional, we consume too much fuel or substance. Therefore, rest and relaxation are the flip side of the coin of activity. Functional activities should be moderate -- not too much and not too little. If there is too little exercise, form or material substance is not adequately consumed and transformed and starts to accumulate and gunk up the works. If there is too little rest, hyperactivity, be that physical, mental, or emotional, consumes too much substance and overheats the organism leading to burnout. This means that diet on the one hand must be balanced by adequate activity and rest/relaxation on the other.

Fire & Essence

The use of a candle as an analogy is actually quite accurate according to Chinese medical theory. Life is seen in TCM as a series of warm transformations. The root yang of the entire body is called the *ming men zhi huo* or the fire of the gate of life. This life fire is responsible for all activities and transformations in the body. We live only as long as this fire of life burns within us and we are stone cold dead when it burns out irrevocably.

This life fire is associated with or has its material basis in the Chinese idea of the kidneys. In Chinese medicine, the kidneys are the fundamental, first organ. They are called the *xian tian zhi ben* or former heaven root. This means they are the prenatal foundation of the organism, both its form and function. The original source of function is the life fire described above. Whereas the most essential material basis or pure substance is referred to as the *jing* essence or *shen jing* kidney essence.

3

In Chinese medicine, there are two types of *jing* essence. There is *xian tian zhi jing* or former heaven essence. This is innate at birth. We are born with a finite amount of this former heaven essence. It is our endowment from our parents and the universe at large and it is stored in the kidneys. This former heaven essence is supplemented by what is called *hou tian zhi jing* or latter heaven essence. This latter heaven essence is manufactured out of the air we breathe and the food and drink we consume. Nutritive essence derived from food is transformed into qi and blood. Qi empowers function and blood nourishes form. As we move through each day, our activities consume both qi and blood. If, when we go to sleep at night, we have manufactured more qi and blood than we have used that day, this excess is transformed into acquired or latter heaven essence. Some of this latter heaven essence is stored in each of the five major organs of Chinese medicine -- the heart, lungs, spleen, liver, and kidneys. However, the major portion of this acquired essence is stored in the kidneys which then form the Fort Knox of the body.

Every metabolic activity, every transformation within the organism requires both some life fire and some *jing* essence to act as the catalyst and substrate respectively. If there were no acquired essence, we would be just like a candle. We would only be born with so much fuel and that would be used up fairly quickly. However, because latter heaven essence derived from our diet supplements our innate former heaven essence stored in our kidneys, this former heaven essence is capable of lasting a lifetime.

4

Longevity, Diet, & Lifestyle

Chinese medical theory believes that the human organism is built to live 100 years. According to the first chapter of the *Nei Jing,* the premier classic of Chinese medicine, most people have enough *jing* essence to last 5 score years. Barring accidental death or infectious disease, we are designed to last 100 years as long as former heaven essence is not squandered by excessive consumption and as long as latter heaven or acquired essence is manufactured and stored to bolster and slow the use of former heaven essence. Since former heaven essence is manufactured from the food and drink we ingest, it is no wonder why Chinese medical theory places such great importance on proper diet and promoting good digestion. Likewise, since acquired essence is stored in the kidneys at night when we sleep, it is no wonder why proper rest and sleep are important as well.

Former heaven essence is like a patrimony or trust fund we inherent at birth. Latter heaven essence is like money which we save in the bank. It is that part of our daily economy above and beyond our operating expenses. When we store it as acquired *jing* essence, it and our former heaven essence together become our body's capital. It is said in alchemy that it takes gold to make gold and that the more gold one has, the more one can make. When applied to our inner alchemy, our original gold is our *jing* essence, both former and latter heaven. When those two essences are full and abundant, organ function is strong, metabolism is efficient, and we generate a profit each day. Therefore, it takes *jing* to make *jing* and the more *jing* we have, the more we can make. When we age, however, instead of living on our interest, we run a negative daily balance and are forced to dip into our capital. Eventually we consume all our capital and we go bankrupt or die.

5

Essence, Qi & Spirit

It is said in Chinese that *jing* essence (material basis) becomes qi (functional activity) and when qi accumulates it becomes *shen* or spirit. *Shen* means consciousness and mental/emotional activities. Excessive thinking or excessive emotionality consume great stores of qi and, therefore, *jing* essence. That is why the fourth basic foundation of good health is a healthy mental attitude. What is meant by a good attitude in Chinese medicine is spelled out fairly exactly. When the seven emotions -- joy, anger, grief, worry, fear, fright, and melancholy -- are appropriate to their stimuli, these are natural subjective experiences and their experience is the purpose of life. Nonetheless, their experience does consume *jing* essence. *Jing* essence without *shen* or mental activity is meaningless in human terms just as a candle which doesn't shed light is also useless. The consumption of *jing* essence through our conscious experience is what is called in Chinese our *shen ming*. *Ming* means brilliance or light. *Jing* essence's purpose is to be transformed into the light of consciousness.

It is further said in Chinese that *shen* should apprehend emptiness and that this apprehension should also be reduced to nothingness. This gets a little abstruse but is worth everyone's understanding, patient and practitioner alike. The apprehension of emptiness means that through one's life experiences one understands that nothing, whether internally experienced or externally existent is permanent or real. If one feels any experience all the way to its depth, it becomes empty. All experiences are reducible to an essential emptiness. Not only are they fleeting but they are of a single, inexpressible, indescribable taste. No matter whether one experiences joy or anger, fear or sadness, these mental/emotional experiences are

6

evanescent and in no way alter or affect the innate nature of the *shen* spirit.

When one understands that the *shen* is inviolable, essentially unharmable, and indestructible, one's experience, whether of good or bad, becomes like a movie projected on a screen. The movie is not the screen and no matter what drama is enacted on the screen, the screen is not harmed or affected. If one can apprehend this, then, in Chinese, one can say that spirit apprehends the essential emptiness of experience. However, if one then becomes attached to this concept of emptiness, that itself can cause an obstruction to the free flow of reality. Therefore, it is further said that emptiness must also be understood as nothingness or no-thing-ness. When one does, this is the absolute good mental attitude which is ultimately healthy.

Deepak Chopra, in *Quantum Healing*, has discussed the therapeutic importance of apprehending this state of absolute emptiness which is uncolored by one's passing and everchanging emotions, thoughts, and sensations. Ironically, this apprehension is in part dependent upon the consumption of *jing* essence. It is a fundamental axiom that *jing* essence is consumed by the aging process and that the signs and symptoms of aging are the signs and symptoms of the kidneys becoming empty and the *jing* becoming insufficient. However, this process results in experiences, and if one has enough experiences and also has enough consciousness to reflect deeply on those experiences, one will understand that, no matter how many times one has been happy or sad, in pleasure or in pain, essentially it has not indelibly colored nor permanently altered one's essential being. This is the wisdom that hopefully comes with old age. It is the wisdom of spontaneous non-attachment, equipoise, naturalness, and the willingness to let things be.

We all get old and we all die. We all experience pain as well as pleasure. These are inevitable. When we fail to recognize the naturalness of this condition and rather take it as a personal affront or attack, we run after pleasure and its means in order to avoid suffering at all cost. Paradoxically, this ceaseless running towards and running away consumes *jing* essence and causes the very disease, suffering, and death we seek to avoid. It is transcendence of this rat-race which the wisdom of the East posits as a good, healthy mental attitude.

Because of the above interrelationships between *jing*, qi and *shen*, it is easy to see why diet, exercise, rest, and the development of such a good, healthy attitude are so important to achieving and maintaining good health. This book focuses on dietary therapy. That does not mean that diet is more important than the other three. The diseases of this time are due to a lack of wisdom in all four of these crucial areas. The contemporary Western diet, although it shows signs of improving, is basically ignorant. We tend to be too sedentary at the same time as being too mentally and emotionally stressed. And few of us can be said to have gained a mature mental equipoise.

It is relatively simple to say that one should get enough exercise and rest. And although Buddhists, Daoists, and Conficianists have filled libraries on how to achieve a good mental attitude, this is not something that can be well conveyed in a book. Diet, on the other hand, is both complex and seemingly open to a great deal of contradiction and confusion. It is also something which can be written about simply and clearly.

The Basic Healthy Diet

The Process of Digestion

I n Chinese, the digestive system is called the *xiao hua xi tong*. The words *xi tong* simply mean system but the words *xiao* and *hua* are more pregnant with meaning. *Xiao* means to disperse and *hua* means to transform. In Chinese medicine, digestion equals the dispersion of pure substances to be retained and impure substances to be excreted after these have undergone transformation. Therefore, the digestive tract is called the *xiao hua dao* or pathway of dispersion and transformation. In TCM we mostly describe the process of digestion in terms of the functions of the Chinese stomach and spleen. Once one understands the functions of the stomach/spleen according to TCM theory, Chinese dietary theory becomes very clear and logical.

Three Burners

The stomach and spleen are a yin yang pair. The stomach is one of the six hollow bowels and is relatively yang. The spleen is one of the five solid organs and is relatively yin. The stomach's function is to receive food and liquids and to "rotten and ripen" these. In Chinese medicine, the stomach is likened to a pot on a fire. As mentioned in the previous chapter, all physiological transformations in Chinese medicine are warm transformations. The body is seen as three alchemical retorts. These are called *jiao* or burners. There is an upper burner containing the heart and lungs, a middle burner containing the stomach and spleen, and a lower burner containing the kidneys, intestines, liver, and reproductive organs.

The Stomach as a Pot

The stomach is the pot of the middle burner and the spleen is both the fire under this pot and the distillation mechanism to which this pot is attached. Just as a mash rottens and ripens in a pot, so foods and liquids rotten and ripen within the stomach. In Chinese medical terms, this means that, as foods and liquids rotten and ripen, the pure and impure parts of these foods and liquids are separated or come apart. It is then the spleen's function to distill or drive off upwards the purest parts of foods and liquids, sending the pure part of foods up to the lungs and the pure part of liquids up to the heart. The pure part of foods or the five flavors become the basis for the creation of qi (pronounced chee) or vital energy within the lungs. The pure part of liquids becomes the basis for the creation of blood within the heart. The sending up of the pure part of the foods and liquids by the spleen is called ascension of the clear.

The stomach then sends down the impure part of foods to be further transformed by the large intestine and the impure parts of liquids to be further transformed by the small intestine. In Chinese medicine, the large intestine's function is to reabsorb the pure part of the impure foods or solids. This becomes the postnatal or latter heaven fuel for kidney yang or the life fire. The small intestine's function is to reabsorb the pure part of the impure parts of liquids. This is transformed into the body's

10

thick liquids, such as cerebrospinal and intra-articular fluids, and nourishes postnatally kidney yin. The large intestine conducts the impure of the impure solids down and out of the body as feces. The small intestine conducts the impure of the impure liquids to the bladder from whence they are excreted as urine. This sending down of the impure part of foods and liquids initiated by the stomach is called the descention of the turbid.

Therefore, in Chinese medicine, digestion is spoken of as the separation of pure (*qing*) and impure or turbid (*zhuo*). This separation is dependent upon the *qi hua* or energy transformation of the middle burner or stomach/spleen and upon the spleen qi's ability to transport or *yun* foods and fluids. Hence, Chinese spleen function is summed up in the two words *yun* (transportation) and *hua* (transformation). *Yun hua* is the older, more traditional form of the modern term *xiao hua*.

The analogy of the cooking pot is very important. It is said in Chinese that the stomach fears or has an aversion to dryness. In other words, stomach function is dependent upon the creating of a mash or soup in its cauldron or pot. It is also said in Chinese that the spleen fears dampness. Since spleen function is likened to a fire under a pot distilling the essence from the mash held in the stomach, it is easy to understand that too much water or dampness can douse or injure that fire.

Using this analogy, it is simple and crucial to understand that the digestive process, according to Chinese medicine, consists of first creating a 100° soup in the stomach, remembering that body temperature is 98.6° F. Whatever facilitates the creation of such a 100° soup in the stomach benefits digestion and whatever impedes or impairs the creation of a 100° soup in the stomach impedes or impairs digestion. This is basically true

11

even from a Western medical perspective. Most of the insights and principles of Chinese dietary theory and therapy are logical extensions of this commonsense and irrefutable truth.

The Implications of This Process:

1. Cooked *vs.* Raw Foods

First of all, TCM suggests that most people, most of the time, should eat mostly cooked food. Cooking is predigestion on the outside of the body to make food more easily digestible on the inside. By cooking foods in a pot on the outside of the body, one can initiate and facilitate the stomach's rottening and ripening in its pot on the inside of the body. Cold and raw foods require that much more energy to transform them into warm soup within the pot of the stomach. Since it takes energy or qi to create this warmth and transformation, the net profit from this transformation is less. Whereas, if one eats cooked foods at room temperature at least or warm at best, less spleen qi is spent in the process of digestion. This means that the net profit of digestion, *i.e.*, qi or energy, is greater.

The idea that eating cooked food is more nutritious than raw food flies in the face of much modern Western nutritional belief. Because enzymes and vitamins are destroyed by cooking, many people think it is healthier to eat mostly raw, uncooked foods. This makes seeming sense only as long as one confuses gross income with net profit. When laboratory scientists measure the relative amounts of cooked and raw foods, they are not taking into account these nutrients' post-digestive absorption.

Let's say that a raw carrot has 100 units of a certain vitamin or

12

nutrient and that a cooked carrot of the same size has only 80 units of that same nutrient. At first glance, it appears that eating the raw carrot is healthier since one would, theoretically, get more of that nutrient that way. However, no one absorbs 100% of any available nutrient in a given food. Because the vitamins and enzymes of a carrot are largely locked in hard to digest cellulose packets, when one eats this raw carrot, they may actually only absorb 50% of the available nutrient. The rest is excreted in the feces. But when one eats the cooked carrot, because the cooking has already begun the breakdown of the cellulose walls, one may absorb 65% of the available nutrient. In this case, even though the cooked carrot had less of this nutrient to begin with, net absorption is greater. The body's economy runs on gross, not net. It is as simple as that. Of course, we are talking about light cooking, and not reducing everything to an overcooked, lifeless mush.

This is why soups and stews are so nourishing. These are the foods we feed infants and those who are recuperating from illness. The more a food is like 100° soup, the easier it is for the body to digest and absorb its nutrients. The stomach/spleen expend less qi and, therefore, the net gain in qi is greater. This is also why chewing food thoroughly before swallowing is so important. The more one chews, the more the food is macerated and mixed with liquids, in other words, the more it begins to look like soup or a stew.

2. Cold Food & Liquids

As a corollary of this, if we drink or eat chilled, cold, or frozen foods or drink iced liquids with our meals, we are only impeding the warm transformation of digestion. Cold obviously negates heat. And water puts out fire. This does not mean that such food and liquids are never digested, but it does mean that often they are not digested well. In Chinese medicine, if the stomach/spleen fail to adequately transport and transform foods and liquids, a sludge tends to accumulate just as it might in an incompletely combusting automobile engine. This sludge is called stagnant food and dampness in Chinese medicine.

3. Dampness & Phlegm

If the solid portions of food are jam-packed into the stomach or their digestion is impaired by cold and chilled foods and liquids or if too many hard to digest foods are eaten, stagnant food may accumulate in the stomach. The stomach tries all the harder to burn these off and becomes like a car stuck in overdrive. It becomes hotter in an attempt to burn off the accumulation. This often results in the stomach becoming chronically overheated. This, in turn, causes the stomach to register hunger which, in Chinese medicine, is a sensation of the stomach's heat. This hunger then results in eating more and more and a vicious loop is created. Overeating begets stagnant food which begets stomach heat which reinforces overeating. Further, persistent stomach heat may eventually waste stomach yin or fluids causing a chronic thirst and preference for cold drinks and chilled foods.

If the liquid portions of food and drink jam the transporting and transforming functions of the spleen, what is called the *qi ji* or qi mechanism in Chinese, these may accumulate as dampness. This plethora of water inhibits the spleen qi's warm transforming function in the same way that water inhibits or douses fire. Over time, this accumulated dampness may mix with stagnant food and congeal into phlegm which further gunks up the entire system and retards the flow of qi and blood throughout the body.

Different people's digestion burns hotter than others'. Those with a robust constitution and strong *ming men* or fire of life tend to have a strong digestion. These people can often eat more in general and more chilled, frozen, hard to digest foods without seeming problems. Likewise, everyone's metabolism runs at different temperatures throughout the year. During the summer when it is hot outside, we generally can eat cooler foods and should drink more liquids. However, even then, we should remember that *everything* that goes down our gullet must be turned into 100° soup before it can be digested and assimilated.

4. Post-Digestive Temperature

In Chinese medicine, there is an important distinction made between the cold physical temperature of a food or drink and a food or drink's post-digestive temperature. Post-digestive temperature refers to a particular food or drink's net effect on the body's thermostat. Some foods, even when cooked, are physiologically cool and tend to lower the body's temperature either systemically or in a certain organ or part. In Chinese medicine, every food is categorized as either cold, cool, neutral, warm, or hot. Most foods are cool, neutral, or warm and, in general, we should mostly eat neutral and warm foods since our body itself is warm. Life is warm. During the winter or in colder climes, it is important to eat warmer foods, but during the summer we can and should eat cooler foods. However, this mostly refers to the post-digestive temperature of a food.

If one eats ice cream in the summer, the body at first is cooled by the ingestion of such a frozen food. However, its response

15

is to increase the heat of digestion in order to deal with this cold insult. Inversely, it is a common custom in tropical countries to eat hot foods since the body is provoked then to sweat as an attempt to cool itself down. In China, mung bean soup and tofu are eaten in the summer because both these foods tend to cool a person down post-digestively. If we are going to eat cold and frozen foods and drink iced, chilled liquids, it is best that these be taken between meals when they will not impede and retard the digestion of other foods.

Many Westerners are shocked to think that cold and frozen foods are inherently unhealthy since they have become such an ubiquitous part of our contemporary diet. However, chilled, cold, and frozen foods and liquids are a relatively recent phenomenon. They are dependent upon refrigeration in the marketplace, refrigeration during transportation, and refrigeration in the home. Such mass access to refrigeration is largely a post World War II occurrence. That means that, in temperate zones, people have only had widespread access to such foods and drinks for less than 50 years. 50 years is not even a blink on the human evolutionary scale.

5. Dampening Foods

Not only do foods have an inherent post-digestive temperature but different foods also tend to generate more or less body fluids. Therefore, in Chinese medicine, all foods can be described according to how damp they are, meaning dampening to the human system. Because the human body is damp, most foods are somewhat damp. We need a certain amount of dampness to stay alive. Dampness in food is yin in that dampness nourishes substance which is mostly wet and gushy. However, some foods are excessively dampening, and, since it

16

is the spleen which avers dampness, *excessively* damp foods tend to interfere with digestion.

According to Chinese five phase theory, dampness is associated with earth. Fertile earth is damp. The flavor of earth according to Chinese five phase correspondence theory is sweet. The sweet flavor is inherently damp and also is nutritive. In Chinese medical terms, the sweet flavor supplements the qi and blood. Qi is energy or vital force and blood in this case stands for all body fluids. Therefore, the sweeter a food or liquid is, the more damp it tends to be.

When one looks at a Chinese medical description of various foods, one is struck by the fact that almost all foods are somewhat sweet and also supplement qi and blood. On reflection, this is obvious. We eat to replenish our qi and blood. Therefore it is no wonder most foods are somewhat sweet. All grains, most vegetables, and most meats eaten by humans are sweet no matter what other of the five flavors they may also be. This sweetness in the overwhelming majority of foods humans regularly eat becomes evident the more one chews a food.

A modicum of sweetness supplements the body's qi and blood. It is this flavor which gathers in the spleen and provides the spleen with its qi. However, excessive sweetness has just the opposite effect on the spleen. Instead of energizing the spleen, it overwhelms and weakens it. This is based on the Chinese idea that yang when extreme transforms into yin and *vice versa*. When the spleen becomes weak, it craves sweetness since that is the flavor which strengthens it when consumed in moderate amounts. However, if this craving is indulged in with concentrated sweets, such as sugar, this only further weakens the spleen and harms digestion. Thus, another pathological loop is forged in many people.

Going back to dampness, the sweet flavor engenders dampness and the sweeter a food is the more dampening it is. According to Chinese medicine, this tendency is worsened when the sweet flavor is combined with sour. Therefore, Chinese medicine identifies a number of especially dampening foods. These include such sweet and sour foods as citrus fruits and juices and tomatoes, such concentrated sweets as sugar, molasses, and honey, and such highly nutritious foods as wheat, dairy products, nuts, oils, and fats.

Highly nutritious foods are those which have more *wei* than qi. All foods are a combination of qi and *wei*. In this context, qi means the light, airy, aromatic and yang part of a food. Whereas, *wei*, literally meaning taste, refers to a food's heavier, more substantial, more nourishing, yin aspects. Highly nutritious foods, such a dairy products, meats, nuts, eggs, oils, and fats are strongly capable of supplementing the body's yin fluids and substances. However, in excess, they generate a superabundance of body fluids which become pathologic dampness. Although to some this may appear a paradox, it has to do with healthy yin in excess becoming evil or pathological yin or dampness, phlegm, and turbidity.

It is also easy to see that certain combinations are even worse than their individual constituents. Ice cream is a dietary disaster. It is too sweet, too creamy, and too cold. Ice cream is a very, very dampening food. Pizza is a combination of tomato sauce, cheese, and wheat. All of these foods tend to be dampening and this effect is made even worse if greasy additions, such as pepperoni and sausage, are added. Tomato sauce bears a few more words. It is the condensed nutritive substances of a number of tomatoes. Therefore it can be especially dampening.

In the same way, drinking fruit juices can be very dampening.

18

Fruit and vegetable juices are another relatively modern addition to the human diet. Prior to the advent of refrigeration as discussed above, juices would turn into wine or vinegar within days. Therefore, when they were available in traditional societies, they were an infrequent treat. Now we have access to tropical fruits and juices thanks to refrigeration and interstate and intercontinental transportation. However, we should bear in mind that we would not eat 4-6 oranges in a single sitting nor every day. When we drink a glass of orange juice, tomato juice, apple juice, or carrot juice, that is exactly what we are doing. We are drinking the nutritive essence of not one but a number of fruits or vegetables. This over-nutrition typically results in the formation of pathogenic dampness and phlegm.

Meats, because they are so nutritious, or supplement qi and blood so much, also tend to be damp in the same way. The fatter and richer a meat is, the more it tends to generate dampness within the body. Amongst the common domestic mammalian meats, pork is the dampest with beef coming in second. Therefore, it is important not to eat too much meat and especially not greasy, fatty meats. Most people do fine on 2 ounces of meat 3-4 times per week.

On the other hand, eating only poultry and fish is not such a good idea either. Everything in this world has its good and bad points. Poultry and fish tend to be less dampening and phlegmatic, it is true, but chicken, turkey, and shellfish tend to be hot. If one eats only these meats, they run the risk of becoming overheated. I have seen this happen in clinical practice. From a Western scientific point of view, we can also say that eating too much fish may result in mercury accumulation and toxicity and overeating commercial chicken may result in too much estrogen and exposure to salmonella food-poisoning. Chinese medicine sees human beings as omnivores and suggests that a person should eat widely and diversely on the food chain.

The Basic Healthy Diet

Therefore, to sum up the traditional wisdom of Chinese dietary theory, humans should mostly eat vegetables and grains with small amounts of everything else. We should mostly eat cooked and warm food which is not too sweet, not too greasy or oily, and not too damp. In addition, we should eat moderately and chew well. It is healthful to drink a teacup of warm water or a warm beverage with meals. This facilitates the formation of that 100° soup. But it is unhealthy to drink or eat chilled, cold, and frozen drinks and foods with meals.

In general, I would emphasize that most Americans do not eat enough vegetables. It is easy to load up on breads, grains, and cereals but not as easy to eat plenty of freshly cooked vegetables. Grains, like meat and dairy products, are highly nutritious but heavy and relatively more difficult to digest. If overeaten they can cause accumulation of dampness and phlegm. In Asia, Daoists and Buddhists interested in longevity emphasized vegetables over grains and even modern Chinese books on geriatrics counsel that more vegetables should be eaten.

Amongst the grains, rice holds an especially healthy place. Because it promotes diuresis, it tends to leech off excessive dampness. Other grains, in comparison, tend to produce dampness as a by-product of their being so nutritious. This ability of rice to help eliminate dampness through diuresis becomes more important the more other dampening foods one eats.

20

Flavors & Spices

As said at the beginning of this chapter, the purest part of foods are the five flavors. These are sweet, salty, bitter, pungent, and sour. Chinese medicine also recognizes a sixth flavor called bland. Each of the five flavors corresponds to one of the five phases and, therefore, tends to accumulate and have an inordinate effect on one of the five major organs of Chinese medicine. Just as overeating sweet injures the spleen, overeating salt injures the kidney, overeating sour injures the liver, and overeating spicy foods injures the lungs. I know of no one who overeats bitter food. A little bitter flavor is good for the heart and stomach. In general, although most food is sweet, one should eat a modicum of all the other flavors. Overeating any one flavor will tend to cause an imbalance in the organs and tissues associated with that flavor according to five phase correspondence.

Most spices are pungent or acrid and warm to hot. These spices aid digestion when eaten in moderate amounts. As discussed above, the digestive process is like an alchemical distillation. The middle burner fire of the stomach/spleen cooks and distills foods and liquids driving off their purest parts. To have good digestion means to have a healthy digestive fire. Moderate use of pungent, warm spices aids digestion by strengthening the middle burner fire.

That is why traditional cultures found the use of pepper, cardamom, cinnamon, ginger, nutmeg, mace, and cloves so salutary. These spices contain a high proportion of qi to *wei* and so help yang qi transform and distill yin substance, dampness, and fluids. On the other hand, when eaten to excess, such spices can cause overheating of the stomach and drying out of stomach fluids, and remember, the stomach does not like to be dry. Therefore, a moderate use of such spices is good for the spleen but their overuse is bad for the stomach and lungs.

A Return to a More Traditional Diet

What this all adds up to is a diet very similar to the Pritikin diet or Macrobiotics. Both these dietary regimes suggest that the bulk of one's diet be composed of complex carbohydrates and vegetables and that one get plenty of fiber and less animal proteins, refined sugars, oils, and fats. This is very much the traditional diet of all people living in temperate climates the world round. This is also very much like what our great grandparents ate.

100 years ago, most people only ate meat once or twice a week. Mostly they ate grains and vegetables. Because they did not have refrigeration, they ate mostly what was in season and what could be stored in root cellars and through pickling, salting, and drying. One hundred years ago, sugar was too expensive for most people to afford more than a tiny bit per year. Likewise, oils and fats were relatively precious commodities and were not eaten in large quantities. Those oils which were available were pressed from flax, hemp, sesame seeds, or were derived from fish oil, lard, and butter. They were not the heavily hydrogenated tropical oils which are so frequently used in commercial food preparation today.

It was also a well-known fact of life 100 years ago that rich people who ate too well and exercised too little were more prone to chronic health problems than those who lived a more spartan and rigorous life. If one looks at the cartoons of the 18th and 19th centuries, one frequently sees the overweight nobleman with the enlarged and gouty toe. Likewise, the

Chinese medical classics contain numerous stories of doctors treating rich patients by getting them to do some physical work and to eat simpler, less rich food. Gerontologists today have noted the fact that those ethnic groups who tend to produce a large proportion of centenarians, such as the Georgians, the Hunzakuts, and certain peoples in the Peruvian Andes, all eat a low animal protein, low fat, high fiber diet.

The Modern Western Diet

The modern Western diet which we take so much for granted is mostly a product of post World War II advances in technology and transportation. Until after World War II, mass refrigeration and interstate transportation did not allow for everyone to buy a half gallon of fresh orange juice anytime of the year at an affordable price nor to keep a half gallon of ice cream (or now frozen yogurt) in their home freezer. In addition, special interest advertising has fostered erroneous ideas about the healthfulness of many of these "new" foods. We have been so bombarded by tv commercials extolling the healthful benefits of orange juice that we seldom remember that these are partisan propaganda bought and paid for by commercial growers who depend upon the sale of their product to turn a profit.

The modern Western diet is a relatively recent aberration in the history of human diet. It is an experiment which has largely run its course as more and more people as well as governmental agencies come to the conclusion that so much of what we take for granted these days as a normal diet is really not healthy. Just as we are now realizing as a society that smoking is bad for the health, likewise we are also now coming to realize that too much sugar, fats, oils, and animal protein are

23

also not good for the health nor conducive to longevity.

Pesticides, Preservatives, & Chemicals

Traditional Chinese Medicine has, in the past, not said anything about pesticides, preservatives, and chemical additives because these things were not known until relatively recently. However, poisoning is a TCM cause of disease listed in the *bu nei bu wai yin* category of neither internal nor external etiologies. All the evidence suggests that eating food which is contaminated by pesticides, preservatives, and chemical dyes and additives is also not good for long term health and well being. Therefore, it is advisable to eat food which is as free from these as possible. That means organic produce and grains and organically grown meat. These are becoming increasingly more common and available.

Wrecked Foods

Since Chinese medicine says that the qi comes from the purest of the pure part of foods, the *xian* or flavor/aroma, Chinese dietary theory also suggests that food should be freshly made and eaten within 24 hours. As food becomes stale, it loses its aroma and its ability to supplement qi is directly proportional to this aroma. Food which is stale is called wrecked food in Chinese. The implication is that, although the substance is still there, the *xian*, aroma, or qi is gone. Such wrecked foods tend to be more dampening and phlegmatic.

I f one follows the above Chinese dietary guidelines, one will eat nutritiously and well. One will be supplemented by their food and not unduly harmed by it. Such a moderate, commonsense diet is one of the four foundations of good health. This diet is more or less appropriate to everyone living in a temperate climate. Patients suffering from specific diseases may require various individualized modifications of the above outlined regime. However, because whether in sickness or health the process of digestion is essentially the same, this is the healthy diet for the majority of people. In the following chapter, we will discuss specific modifications for the most common groups of imbalance described by TCM. Yet even these modifications are based on this same commonsense approach to food and eating.

THE PILL & STAGNANT BLOOD

THE SIDE EFFECTS OF ORAL CONTRACEPTIVES ACCORDING TO TRADITIONAL CHINESE MEDICINE

Since 1960 when birth control pills were first introduced, they have become a fact of modern life. As an American practitioner of Traditional Chinese Medicine specializing in gynecology, I find use of the Pill at some point in my patients' lives is almost 100%. Because this is such a universal factor in my patients' medical histories, I have had, by necessity, to come to some conclusions regarding the Pill's TCM functions and effects. Although Dr. James W. Long lists 28 different kinds of combined estrogen/progestin oral contraceptives available in the United States manufactured by six different companies[1], I think it is possible to describe the TCM functions and effects of the Pill as if these were a single traditional Chinese, polypharmacy formula.

The intended therapeutic effect of combined oral contraceptives is to prevent pregnancy through the suppression of ovulation. Traditional Chinese Medicine, however, has no theory of ovulation *per se*. Traditional Chinese doctors are limited to information gathered only by our traditional Four Methods of Diagnosis (*Si Zhen*). These are Inspection (*Wang Zhen*), Olfaction/Auscultation (*Wen Zhen*), Palpation (*Qie Zhen*), and Interrogation (*Wen Zhen*). Inspection is limited to only that which can be seen with the unaided, naked eye. Since the ovum is not visible amidst the menstruate by the naked eye, traditional Chinese doctors have no concept of ovum in our

medicine. ;Chinese doctors know that a man must ejaculate in a woman's vagina for conception to occur. We also know that a woman cannot become pregnant before menarche, a woman bleeds from her vagina monthly, and that this bleeding stops during pregnancy and at menopause when she becomes infertile. The only thing other than leukorrhea and babies which the Chinese doctor knows that comes from the vagina is Blood. Therefore, traditional doctors throughout Asia have believed, and pragmatically so, that conception takes place when the woman's Blood combines with the man's Reproductive Essence (*Sheng Zhi Zhi Jing* or sperm) within her *Xue She* or Blood Chamber.

The modern TCM practitioner knows that birth control pills make a woman infertile. This is common knowledge and can be ascertained through questioning. However, the Western medical explanation of how this is effected cannot be plugged into our conceptual methodology since we have no such concept as the ovum, nor can this concept be added to our system without rending its conceptual fabric. According to TCM theory, there are basically two broad categories of *Bing Ji* or Disease Mechanism accounting for infertility. These are 1) Insufficiency of Blood and 2) Stagnation of Blood. In the first case, there simply is not enough Blood in the Blood Chamber to unite with the man's Reproductive Essence. This can be due to hypofunction of the Spleen, Heart, or Kidneys, the three Chinese Organs which *Hua* or transform the Blood. In the second case, although there may be sufficient Blood, it is blocked and does not flow properly. Therefore, it cannot unite with the man's *Sheng Zhi Zhi Jing*. Factors causing Stagnation of Blood in a woman's Lower Burner include Cold, Liver Qi Congestion, Stagnant Heat, Phlegm Dampness, and trauma.

By looking at the total constellation of effects that the Pill has on women, I think it is possible to say that oral contraceptives induce iatrogenic infertility by causing Stagnation. This

becomes apparent when we look for the common *Bing Ji* for
the Pill's various side effects. These side effects include those
which are considered "natural, expected, and unavoidable" and
those which are "unusual, unexpected, and infrequent".[2] In the
first category we find edema, weight gain, mid-cycle or breakthrough bleeding, change in menstrual flow (usually becoming
scanter), absence of menstrual flow, and an increased tendency
to yeast infections. In the second category are skin rashes,
itching, and hives; headache, nervous tension, and irritability;
accentuation of migraine headaches; nausea, vomiting, and
bloating; breast enlargement, tenderness, and secretion; tannish
pigmentation of the face; and reduced tolerance to contact
lenses. More serious and even life-threatening adverse
reactions include muscle and joint pains, thrombophlebitis,
pulmonary embolism, stroke, high blood pressure, coronary
embolism, retinal thrombosis, hepatitis with jaundice, emotional
depression (which may be severe), formation of liver neoplasms,
and gallbladder disease.

Although this litany of woes is long and seemingly diverse, all
these may be explained in TCM terms as complications of
Stagnation. Above I said that infertility is due to either Insufficient or Stagnant Blood. However, that was a bit of an over-
simplification in my attempt to clarify the Blood's pivotal role
in the TCM theory of fertility. There are Six Stagnations in
Chinese medicine and all six are mutually promoting. They are
Stagnant Qi, Stagnant Blood, Stagnant Food, Stagnant Heat,
Stagnant Dampness, and Stagnant Phlegm. But, within these
six, the first two are the two most discussed vis a vis menstruation and conception. Qi controls the Blood. In particular, this
means that Qi transports, circulates, or moves the Blood. The
Blood is the mother of the Qi. That means the Blood is the
Root of the Qi, its substrate and foundation. Therefore, Qi
Stagnation may lead to Blood Stagnation and Blood Stagnation
may lead to Qi Stagnation. Since they both flow together, if
one gets stuck, so will the other over time.

In the case of birth control pills, I believe this Stagnation begins with Liver Qi Congestion. It is the Liver which stores the Blood. The *Chong Mai*, the Vessel which controls menstruation and conception, is called the Sea of Blood and the Liver plays an important role in regulating this Vessel. The Liver's job is to store sufficient Blood so that menstruation and conception can occur *and* also to ensure this Blood's unhindered circulation. The Liver maintains the patency of Qi flow and, therefore, Blood flow of the entire organism, but it especially is responsible for the patency of circulation within the Lower Burner. All of the side effects of birth control pills can be explained as stemming from Liver Qi Congestion.

Nausea, vomiting, and bloating as a syndrome suggest Liver Qi invading the Stomach. Breast enlargement and tenderness are also primarily due to Liver Qi according to TCM.[3] Migraine headaches are usually a combination in women of Ascending Liver Yang and Blood Deficiency. First, the Liver Qi congests. This repletion of Qi causes exhaustion or evaporation of the Blood. When this Qi accumulates sufficiently, it vents upward coming apart from its foundation, the Blood, usually along the course of the *Shao Yang*. This causes headaches and neck tension in general and migraines in particular. Irritability is a well-known and common symptom of all Liver Qi originating or complicated scenarios. Since the eyes are the aperture of the Liver and since Liver Qi typically transforms into Heat which rises upward, eye irritation is easily understood. Retention of fluid and weight gain have to do with Liver Qi invading the Spleen and effecting that Organ's ability to *Yun* and *Hua* Fluids. Breakthrough bleeding is usually due to Depressive Heat causing the Blood to run recklessly out of its Channels, remembering the Chinese character for Channel (*Jing*) is the same as for menstruation. Scant periods are due to this Heat's evaporating the Blood. Amenorrhea may occur if either the Blood is wasted to the point where there is insufficient Blood to have a period or if the Qi Congestion leads to Blood

Stagnation with Blood Deficiency. Skin rashes are mostly due to Liver Heat, while itching is a species of Internal stirring of Wind due to Blood Deficiency. Increased tendency to vaginitis is also due to Transformative Depressive Heat in the Liver, remembering that it is the Liver Channel which irrigates the genitalia. Depression is another classic Liver symptom and even tannish pigmentation of the face has a Liver connection. In Chinese medicine, this is called *Huang E Ban*. Its Disease Mechanism is Spleen Deficiency causing Blood Deficiency complicated by Liver Wind and Heat[4]. This then causes Stagnation in the *Sun Luo* Above which gives the face a darker than normal color.

The more serious adverse effects of the Pill likewise participate in this Liver Qi/Blood Stagnation connection. Muscle and joint pain in women with a history of using the Pill is often either/or a combination of Stagnant Blood and Blood Insufficiency failing to nourish the *Jin* Sinews and *Mai* Vessels.[5] Thrombophlebitis, pulmonary embolism, and coronary thrombosis all are indicative of Stagnant Blood. In these cases, Stagnant Qi over time has resulted in Stagnant Blood. Stroke or CVA, on the other hand, is due to Liver Qi or Transformative Fire engendering Wind which gives rise to *Zhong Feng* or Windstroke. In women, there is a *Bing Ji* for high blood pressure due to Stagnant Blood injuring the *Chong*.[6] Retinal thrombosis suggests Stagnant Blood if there is pain and visible hemorrhage or exhaustion of Liver Blood if there is only sudden loss or impairment of vision. Hepatitis with jaundice is due to Depressive Liver Qi when due in turn to oral contraceptives. Whereas, abdominal tumors in the hypochondrium are a classic symptom of Stagnant Blood due to Stagnant Liver Qi. And cholecystitis/cholelithiasis also may be due not only to Damp Heat in the Gallbladder but also to Stagnant Liver Qi and Stagnant Blood.[7]

Because women who begin taking oral contraceptives have

various already pre-existing conditions, how any given woman will react to the Pill will also vary. For instance, some women with dysmenorrhea before taking the Pill experience its cessation when on the Pill. Typically, these women also experience a diminution in menstrual flow when on the Pill. When they go off the Pill, if the oral contraceptives have not caused a permanent worsening of their condition, they usually will also experience a resumption of their period pain. In such cases, the Pill causes more Stagnation of Blood and so less flow. It must be remembered that Stagnation of Blood impairs the creation of fresh or new Blood. On the Pill, there is not enough volume of flow with the period to experience the pressure of dysmenorrhea. When the Pill is suspended, the circulation is relatively freed and the Blood, therefore, may become more in volume. Since there is still Stagnation, this increased flow and volume causes the return of dysmenorrhea.

Other women may not experience any period pain before taking the Pill but have intense dysmenorrhea while on it. In this case, the woman usually does not have significant, pre-existing Stagnation. When she begins oral contraceptives, this causes Stagnation. If her volume of Qi and Blood is relatively full, this Stagnation may be experienced during menstruation as dysmenorrhea. Yet other women may experience the complete cessation of menstruation when taking oral contraceptives with failure to resume menstruating even after discontinuing the Pill. These women usually already have Blood Deficiency which is then severely complicated by Stagnation. In effect, these women are rendered permanently sterile unless treated by Traditional Chinese Medicine in order to disperse Stagnation and tonify the Blood.

Some women are put on the Pill not in order to cause temporary infertility but in order to regulate their period. These women are suffering from what in Chinese medicine is called *Yue Jing Bu Tiao*, Irregular Menstruation. These women may

get their periods either early or late or on no fixed schedule. Because the Pill does make the period come precisely on time, I think that we can also theorize that so-called combined oral contraceptives have a two cycle function. First they Stagnate the Qi (and Blood) to prevent conception. Then they activate the Qi and Blood to promote menstruation. Although they also seem to have their own internal Qi-activating effect, essentially, this artificial stagnation and activation of the Qi and Blood results in Stagnation and Exhaustion of the Blood.

Case History

The following case history is a typical report from a young American woman. The patient was a 22 year old college student. Her major complaint was intense intravaginal burning in response to the presence of semen. There were no sores or inflammation on her external genitalia and internal gynecological examination had likewise revealed no internal sores or inflammation. This burning had begun at 19 years of age. During this same time, she had recurrent yeast infections after each period. These a Western gynecologist had diagnosed as a pH imbalance one year before seeing me. The patient was able to control these infections by douching with distilled water after each period. This young woman had taken the Pill from 14 to 18 years of age and then again from 19 to 1 month before seeing me. During the time she was on the Pill, she also experienced lack of vaginal lubrication during sex which was improving since discontinuing the Pill. When on the Pill, her menstrual cramps were relatively intense every month. She experienced both cramping and stabbing pain and she needed to take a Western painkiller. When she stopped the Pill, her period pain diminished. Also when on the Pill, her periods were excessive in volume and bright red. Premenstrually, she experienced irritability, lower abdominal bloating, and craving

for chocolate. Her tongue was redder than normal with a yellowish fur. Her pulse was slippery and full in the *Cun* and *Guan* positions and wiry in the *Chi*.

My diagnosis was Liver Heat and Stagnation of Qi and Blood. Her Blood was relatively full. The oral contraceptives (in this case Norinyl) had caused intensification of the Stagnation. Because she was young and robust, this Stagnation led to Transformative Heat. Therefore I prescribed *Long Dan Xie Gan Tang* (Dragon Gall Purge Liver Decoction) in its Jade Pharmacy form of Quell Fire, 2 tablets 3 times per day. This was to specifically address her major complaint of vaginal burning with intercourse and ejaculation. I also counselled this young woman that her condition would not be completely rectified until we also subsequently eradicated her dysmenorrhea and PMS. This woman is still undergoing TCM treatment as we work to the Root of her condition.

Conclusion

Happily this woman, although she began the use of oral contraceptives at a very young age, is dealing with the iatrogenic consequences of the Pill also at a relatively very young age. Most of my patients are women in their thirties whose conditions are typically complicated by at least one or more abortions and various venereal and lower abdominal infections treated by various antibiotics, all of which also tend to cause Stagnation of Blood in the Lower Burner.[8] In my opinion, use of oral contraceptives are at least partially responsible for the apparent rise in PMS and endometriosis and infertility in modern women. It is my firm clinical impression and it is also logical according to TCM theory that use of the Pill does predispose a woman to breast, uterine, thyroid, and liver neoplasms. I am afraid that we are going to see an epidemic of these in ten years in the

same women who are experiencing PMS and endometriosis today. Chinese medicine has both the theory and therapy to stop such an epidemic.

Beyond that, Western practitioners of Traditional Chinese Medicine, it seems to me, have an ethical obligation both to perfect our traditional Chinese diagnostic and therapeutic skills and to also extend our theory to cover the full gamut of stimuli which our patients experience. That means describing Western foods, Western drugs, Western herbs, vitamins, minerals, amino acids, etc. all according to the rubric of Chinese medicine. Only if we do that will our medicine truly speak to and address the needs of our patient population. As Jeremy Ross has written in *Zang Fu,*

> The incorrect use, or the side effects of the correct use, of Western medicines and treatments may result in deep and lasting disharmonies of the mind, the emotions, and the physical body. The signs of these drug-induced disharmonies are very common in the West, and can greatly confuse diagnosis. The practitioner must be aware of treatment as a common disease factor, and must assess this possibility in every case.[9]

Chinese medical theory is general enough that it can provide universally valid and pragmatic conclusions about any stimuli from any source if that stimuli creates effects which register according to our Four (Methods of) Diagnosis. Attempting to describe disease factors and stimuli which have not already been described by TCM is a complicated and time-consuming task which requires a high degree of proficiency in Chinese medical theory. It is a task somewhat analogous to Li Shi-zhen's monumental expansion of the *Ben Cao* in the sixteenth century. But, whether difficult or not, it is a task mandated by historical imperative, and a journey of a thousand *Li* begins with the first step.

ENDNOTES

1   Long, James W., *The Essential Guide to Prescription Drugs*, Fourth Edition, Harper & Row, NY, 1985, p. 571

2   Ibid., p. 573-574

3   See Wolfe, Honora Lee, *The Breast Connection, A Laywoman's Guide to the Treatment of Breast Disease by Chinese Medicine*, Blue Poppy Press, Boulder, CO, 1989, for a full discussion of this scenario.

4   Liang Jian-hui, *A Handbook of Traditional Chinese Dermatology*, trans. by Zhang Ting-liang & Bob Flaws, Blue Poppy Press, Boulder, CO, 1988, p. 118-120

5   Ou Yang-yi, *Handbook (of) Differential Diagnosis (&) Treatment*, trans. by C.S. Cheung, Harmonious Sunshine Cultural Center, SF, 1987, p. 77

6   Lu, Henry, *Doctor's Manual of Chinese Medical Diet (2)*, Chinese Foundation of Natural Health, Vancouver, 1981, p. 14

7   Chace, Charles, "Between a Rock and a Hard Place, Treatment of Gall Bladder Disease Using Chinese Herbal Medicine," *Journal of the American College of TCM*, San Fancisco, #3, 1987, p. 18-27

8   Flaws, Bob, "Pelvic Inflammatory Disease (PID)" *Free & Easy, Traditional Chinese Gynecology for American Women*, Blue Poppy Press, Boulder, CO, 1986, p. 37-46

9   Ross, Jeremy, *Zang Fu, The Organ Systems of Traditional Chinese Medicine*, Second Edition, Churchill Livingstone, Edinburgh, 1985, p. 44

Remedial Dietary Therapy

C hinese remedial dietary therapy is based on the foundation of the healthy diet described in the preceding chapter. No matter what the disease or illness, the process of digestion remains the same and, therefore, the overall requirements for diet also remain the same. Because of the interrelationships between the various organs and bowels, qi, blood, and body fluids, yin and yang, and because of the pivotal nature of the middle burner or stomach/spleen, adherence to this basic healthy diet benefits essentially all conditions.

However, within the professional practice of Chinese dietary therapy, there are specific foods and recipes which are prescribed remedially for specific diseases. In fact, the TCM definition of dietary therapy or *yin shi liao fa* is the prescription of particular foods as if they were medicinal substances. In this short layperson's introduction I do not intend to go into these. These specifics should be prescribed by a professional practitioner of TCM. In my own clinical practice I have found that giving patients access to the technical TCM descriptions of individual foods is more confusing than beneficial.

The composition of individualized dietary recipes and the approval or removal of individual foods from a particular patient's diet requires a professionally technical understanding of that person's TCM diagnosis. In turn, the professional practice of TCM requires years of study and deep thought coupled with clinical experience. In my experience, laypersons tend to arrive at incorrect dietary assumptions when they attempt to assess the personal relevance of each individual food from a TCM food materia medica. This is in part because such information is conveyed in a technical vocabulary whose words do not necessarily mean what they do in everyday parlance.

For instance, if one reads that watercress benefits water (as one might in my wife's and my *Prince Wen Hui's Cook*) and does not know that water in Chinese medicine can mean either pathologic dampness or healthy yin, one might wrongly increase their consumption of this food in order to supplement yin. However, because this food is cool, it weakens stomach/spleen yang. Because kidney yin or *jing* is manufactured from the daily excess of qi and blood produced from the products of digestion transformed by the stomach/spleen, such weakening of stomach/spleen function will only tend to compound yin emptiness. This is especially so since the verb *li*, to benefit (or more correctly to disinhibit) means to increase diuresis. Watercress helps to drain yin fluids from the body *via* urination, thus possibly aggravating yin fluid emptiness and dryness in a person suffering from that condition. This is made more complex by the fact that if a person is kidney yin empty or weak, kidney qi may not adequately transform and transport liquids and so, sometimes, such a diuretic medicinal is included as part of an overall treatment plan to nourish and enrich yin and body fluids. This all depends upon the relative proportions of pathologic or evil water *vis a vis* righteous body fluids.

As the lay reader can see, this all gets pretty technical and complicated pretty quickly and such specific recommendations are best left to their professional TCM practitioner. Nonetheless, there are some general recommendations that can be made regarding the appropriate Chinese dietary therapy for some of the most commonly encountered patterns of imbalance. These are spleen emptiness and dampness, liver depression and stomach heat, kidney yin emptiness, and damp heat.

Spleen Emptiness and Dampness

The spleen may become empty or weak due to overfatigue, excessive worry, or overeating sweets and cold, raw foods and drinks. When the spleen becomes weak, its functions of transporting and transforming may become impaired. Typically this results in fluids accumulating in the spleen which are then referred to as pathologic or evil dampness. Once this evil dampness has accumulated in the spleen, it further impairs spleen yang or digestive fire and a vicious circle forms. The spleen is too weak to distil and evaporate or transport and transform this dampness away and this dampness keeps the spleen from recuperating its strength or qi.

This is a commonly encountered problem in clinical practice. Often spleen weakness and dampness begin in infancy with inappropriately scheduled feeding and poor choices in foods for the immature newborn. Mothers should see my *Food, Phlegm, and Pediatric Disease: The Care and Feeding of Infants According to Traditional Chinese Medicine.* Spleen weakness and dampness are especially prevalent amongst Westerners. This is because of our current lack of wisdom regarding the feeding of newborns and infants, our sweet tooth, our overconsumption of fats and oils, our use of wheat as our staple grain (which tends to be damp and cool), and our fondness for raw, cold, and damp foods in general. All these factors contribute to the prevalence of spleen weakness and dampness in the West. Because of the pivotal and absolutely crucial importance of stomach/spleen or middle burner function to the health and well being of the entire organism, such spleen weakness and dampness may cause or complicate innumerable diseases.

If one has been diagnosed by a professional practitioner of TCM as having a weak and/or damp spleen, one should avoid concentrated sweets such as sugar, honey, molasses, and maple syrup. Although some sweets are warm, such as barley malt, and, therefore, not as deleterious to the spleen as, say, white sugar which is cool, still any concentrated sugar can overwhelm the spleen and generate excessive fluids and dampness.

One should minimize their consumption of cold foods. This means foods and drinks which are chilled or frozen. If a food or drink has been stored in the refrigerator, it should be heated up to at least room temperature before being consumed. Person's suffering from spleen weakness and dampness should especially not eat such cold and chilled foods with other foods which would only impair their digestion and absorption. Cold foods also mean energetically cool and cold foods. For instance, lettuce, celery, cucumbers, watermelon, mung beans, buckwheat, seaweeds, mangoes, millet, pear, persimmon, spinach, tomatoes, and wheat are all cool or cold and overconsumption of these foods can chill the middle burner or spleen yang. If these foods are eaten raw or cold, this further worsens their cooling effect.

One should also avoid eating dampening foods and drinking too many liquids with meals. Dampening foods include milk and dairy products, citrus fruits and juices, pineapple juice, tomatoes, sugar and sweets, and fatty, greasy, oily foods. Some persons suffering from spleen dampness may experience constant thirst and may crave liquids. However, this seeming paradox is important to understand. Since fluids are not being transported from the middle burner to the rest of the body in order to moisten and nourish them, these parts of the body may experience thirst or dryness. Yet the more one drinks and floods the spleen with further dampness, the worse and more deeply entrenched this condition becomes. Patients with this diagnosis need to consume less liquids and especially with meals. At first, their thirst and craving for fluids will increase, but, as the body becomes starved for fluids, the spleen will be forced to give up those that are waterlogging it. Typically, the body's wisdom recognizes what must be done and where to get the liquids it needs within 2-3 days.

What this means from the positive point of view is that people with spleen weakness and dampness should eat a lot of cooked vegetables, cooked rice, small amounts of relatively dry animal protein, such as chicken, turkey, and white fish, and a modicum of preferably cooked fruits. In addition, they should use a moderate amount of drying and warming, spleen strengthening spices and seasonings, such as cardamon, black pepper, ginger (both dry and fresh), cinnamon, and nutmeg. They should eat foods which are light and easy to digest. They should eat soups and stews. And they should chew their food thoroughly. In addition, their practitioners may suggest taking digestive enzymes with meals to supplement their stomach/spleen.

Liver Depression, Stomach Heat

This is another extremely common pattern of imbalance here in the West. Liver depression means stagnation of the qi due to the liver's being jammed up and not free flowing. This is mostly due to emotional stress, what in Chinese is called internal injury due to the seven passions. The Chinese liver is in charge of spreading the qi and maintaining its free flow or patency. Any kind of emotional stress can cause stagnation of liver qi but especially anger and frustration or a feeling of being stuck, trapped, or held back.

31

Although liver depression and qi stagnation are primarily due to mental/emotional causes, they are complicated by certain dietary factors. The free flow of stomach/spleen qi is dependent in part on the free flow of liver qi. If one overeats and develops food stagnation in the stomach and intestines, this will impede the free flow of stomach/spleen qi which will, in turn, negatively affect liver qi. Therefore, those with liver qi stagnation should be careful not to overeat or stuff themselves full of heavy, hard to digest foods. In other words, one should not eat a lot of nuts, nut butters, bread, and meat.

When the liver becomes stuck, it also becomes full of qi. Since qi is warm, liver stagnation often becomes hot as well. This is called transformative or stagnant heat. Therefore, it is also important not to eat too many energetically hot foods if one's Chinese liver tends to be stuck or stagnant. This includes hot, spicy, pungent, and acrid foods. Often people with liver stagnation and depression crave such spicy, hot foods since they are qi stimulants and, at least temporarily, resolve the feeling of impatency and depression. However, if the liver is not only stuck but hot, such hot, spicy foods will cause this heat to flare up even more, thus complicating this scenario. Rather, it is better to increase one's exercise, go to funny movies, practice daily deep relaxation, and attempt to solve those problems in one's life that make one feel stuck and frustrated.

Because the liver and the stomach both get their warmth from the fire of the gate of life (the *ming men zhi huo*), if one of these becomes overheated, the other also typically becomes inflamed. This means that liver depression and stagnant heat are often coupled with a hot stomach as well. Because the liver and gallbladder are a yin yang pair, if the liver becomes stuck and overheated, the gallbladder can likewise become unhealthily hot. And all this may be compounded by a damp, weak spleen. In such cases, it is important to avoid alcohol, coffee, greasy, oily foods, fatty meats, and chemicals and preservatives. Although one may have an excessive appetite and crave cold foods and drinks, one needs to exercise some care.

If one is truly excess and has a robust spleen but a hot liver and stomach, one's TCM practitioner may advise eating some cold foods, such as raw lettuce, celery, spinach, tofu, soybean sprouts, mung bean sprouts, radishes, coriander, etc. However, that does not mean that these should be overeaten. The middle burner is still the middle *burner*. One should eat even more freshly cooked vegetables, and especially dark, leafy greens, but one should not go overboard eating all cold, raw foods.

According to the *Nei Jing*, in cases of liver disease, one should first treat the spleen since, according to five phase theory, the spleen will next be affected if it isn't already. A strong, healthy spleen can do a great deal to keep a full, hot liver in check. Therefore, one should follow the general guidelines for supplementing and disinhibiting the spleen in combination with a modicum of cool and cold foods and medicinals for the liver, gallbladder, and stomach.

Often people with a chronically full and stagnant liver will want to know about the do's and don'ts of diet in great detail. They will gravitate towards lists and stringent and exact guidelines detailing every aspect of what they put in their mouths. This tendency is a symptom of this imbalance. Person's with this complaint should recognize this and try to relax more. Ultimately, liver depression and qi stagnation are emotional issues which need to be addressed primarily on that level. If one with such an imbalance becomes fixated on diet, they miss the point of their diagnosis, for in the end, the key piece of advice to such persons is to kick back and relax.

Kidney Yin Emptiness

Life in the West is extremely fast paced. We are flooded with stimuli, are constantly on the go, and we tend to burn our candles from both ends. Due to sex, drugs, and rock n' roll, many of us have prodigally burnt through our yin substance and *jing* essence. Since the Chinese kidneys are the repository of true or righteous yin and essence, this leads to their weakness and emptiness. In Chinese medicine, the aging process is exactly equivalent to the weakening and decline of the kidneys. We can say we are as old as our kidneys are. As one ages, one inevitably consumes yin. Thus one becomes dry and wrinkled, stooped and bent, one's hair goes gray or falls out, one's teeth fall, one's vision and hearing become dim, one's sexual capacity declines, and one's mental brilliance begins to fade. TCM attributes all this to kidney weakness and deficiency.

As we have seen in the preceding chapter, the stomach/spleen get the source of their heat from kidney yang or the fire of of life. Conversely, the essential substances and nutrients digested by the stomach/spleen are transformed into yin essence which then shore up and bolster the kidneys. In addition, the *Nei Jing* says that the *yang ming* or stomach and intestinal function begins to decline at around 35, *before* the kidneys begin their decline.

One of the reasons why many Westerners are prematurely yin empty is that our diet is typically so unsupportive of the stomach/spleen, and the main way to supplement kidney yin dietarily is through strengthening and disinhibiting the spleen. If the spleen is strong and capable of ascending the pure and descending the turbid, an excess of qi and blood is made each day which is converted into *jing* essence to be stored in the kidneys when we sleep. Therefore, people with kidney yin emptiness should, once again, eat the basic middle burner-benefitting diet described above.

Such patients however, can and should eat a bit more meat and animal proteins than others. Most of the foods which Chinese dietary theory identifies as directly supplementing kidney yin are animal meats and organs. This is because we are talking about yin substance which in the human is one's organs, meat, and flesh. Animal meats and organs are made from the same molecules and constituents as our own body, our own substance. Therefore, such animal foods are the most direct way to get the building blocks and constituents of this yin essence.

Chinese eat all sorts of fish and game that most Westerners do not. Seaslugs, jellyfish, abalone, mussels, clams, testicles, kidneys, hearts, livers, brains, all sorts of eggs, turtles, and all the other fleshy exotica of Chinese cuisine are, from a Chinese medical point of view, eaten because they are kidney yin and *jing* essence supplements. However, Chinese doctors also say that these foods should not be overeaten since, because they are so nutritious (*i.e.*, have so much *wei* as compared to qi), they are also dampening, greasy, and hard to digest. Again, the issue is a modicum or moderate amount of these -- more perhaps than someone who is not yin empty but not so much as to complicate one's condition with a lot of phlegm and dampness.

Although lay readers may find it hard at first to understand how a person could be yin empty and also damp and phlegmatic (though both are yin, one is righteous and the other is pathologic), many Americans are just that. It is not uncommon in clinical practice to find persons who are damp, phlegmatic, and obese "on the outside" who are parched and dry "on the inside". From a TCM technical point of view, the words inside and outside are not exactly correct, but hopefully one gets the general picture. For these people, sticking to the basic stomach/spleen diet outlined above is their best possible course of action. They should depend upon the connection between the middle burner and the kidneys and the fact that healthy digestion will automatically result in shoring up depleted yin. This was Li Dong-yuan's approach to treating yin emptiness. Li Dong-yuan was one of the four great masters of internal medicine of the Jin-Yuan Dynasties.

Therefore, persons with kidney yin emptiness and insufficiency should avoid sugars and sweets, alcohol, coffee, and other stimulants, the *excessive* use of dry, pungent, warm, and acrid spices, and should also avoid Nutrasweet and other artificial sweeteners. Clinical experience suggests that these weaken kidney qi. Rather, a person should eat plenty of warm, easy to digest soups and stews, lots of cooked vegetables and grains, and a bit more animal protein than someone else might. As long as a person does not suffer from dampness and phlegm complicating their emptiness and insufficiency, one can eat relatively more wheat and oats which tend to have a lubricating and calming effect.

Damp Heat

The fourth pattern of imbalance which I see most often in clinical practice are various types of damp heat. Most often, the dampness is due to faulty stomach/spleen function. Due to faulty diet, worry, and overfatigue, if the spleen fails to *yun* and *hua* liquids as it should, these, being heavy, have a tendency to seep downwards and collect in the lower part of the body. This dampness impedes the flow of qi wherever it collects. The qi backs up behind the puddled and pooled dampness and, because qi is warm, the area becomes overheated. This heat then become tied up or bound with the dampness and becomes what is called in Chinese medicine *shi re* or damp heat. Technically, this heat may be either full, depressive, or empty heat, but, once it joins with dampness, it is damp heat nonetheless.

Damp heat may manifest as problems with the liver and gallbladder or various inflammatory conditions of the intestines, bladder, and reproductive organs. It can also cause various dermatological or skin diseases. Once damp heat gets established in the lower part of the body, it can be difficult to rid. This is due to dampness' heaviness and turbidity. Chinese medicine says dampness is recalcitrant to treatment. In addition, a certain amount of damp heat typically accumulates as one ages.

Since dampness mostly has its source in the middle burner, once again a common sense, middle burner, stomach/spleen-benefitting diet is important to correct the generation of dampness at its source. Even if the heat in damp heat is empty heat, such an approach will still benefit the situation. In addition, persons with damp heat in the lower burner or lower half of their body should eat somewhat more cooling, diuretic foods. These include Chinese barley or Job's tears, water and other summer melons, watercress, celery, carrots, cranberries, and cucumbers. However, except for the melons and cranberries, these should all be eaten lightly cooked. Because rice is mildly diuretic, it should be the staple grain for those suffering from damp heat in the lower burner. Sweets, chocolate, nuts, ice cream, frozen yogurt, alcohol, greasy, oily, and fatty foods should be avoided. Chinese dietary theory holds that oils and alcohol are especially productive of dampness and heat.

N eophytes when they first get into Chinese medicine tend to be fascinated by all the exotica. There are any number of Chinese dietary books written in Chinese that give Chinese recipes for various health conditions. It can be fun eating day lily flower because Chinese medicine says these are good for sorrow or turtle and sasparilla soup for damp heat and liver/kidney emptiness. But after more than a dozen years studying, eating, and prescribing Chinese foods according to Chinese dietary theory and therapy, I have come to the conclusion that most people do best if they stick to what I have called a basic middle burner, spleen-benefitting diet: warm food cooked fresh and eaten warm, lots of fresh vegetables, lots of grains, some beans, a little animal protein of all sorts and varieties, a moderate consumption of fruits, seeds, and nuts, not much concentrated sweets, oils, or fats, and plenty of fiber. Professional practitioners or other readers interested in the technical TCM descriptions of specific foods are referred to my and Honora Lee Wolfe's *Prince Wen Hui's Cook: Chinese Dietary Therapy* published by Paradigm Publications of Brookline, MA. However, let me reiterate one more time, I believe it is more important to understand the basic wisdom of Chinese dietary theory than get lost in a sea of technical details and Oriental exotica.

Food Allergies

F ood allergies are a common diagnosis amongst Westerners and especially those who seek their health care from so-called alternative practitioners, such as chiropractors, naturopaths, and homeopaths. In Chinese medicine there is no such disease category as food allergies. That is not to say there are no food allergies but that TCM does not categorize the signs and symptoms of such allergies as a distinct disease. In part this is because, in my experience, Chinese are far less prone to food allergies than Westerners. I believe this is so exactly because traditional Chinese dietary sense is so much better in general than contemporary Western dietary sense. Most Chinese know more about the good and bad effects of food and know better how to eat healthfully than most Westerners. Therefore, they have less problems due to eating the wrong foods at the wrong time.

Most food allergies begin in infancy where our current Western lack of nutritional sense is most glaring and apparent. Chinese medical theory states that the child's stomach/spleen or their digestion is immature until at least 6 years of age. When a person is a beginner at something with undeveloped skills and abilities, we normally recognize the need to start off slowly and easily until one develops the requisite skills and abilities. Babies need to be fed beginner's foods. That means mother's milk, watered down cereal soups, mashed, cooked vegetables, and small amounts of animal soups and broths. Instead, we ply our infants with cold fruit juices, raw carrots, apples, oranges, cheese, fried foods and chips, peanut butter, and cold milk and sweetened yogurt out of the refrigerator.

As we have seen in the preceding chapters, such foods are very dampening and relatively hard to digest. These foods may be very nutritious for a grownup with a strong digestion, but they are very difficult to digest for a child below the age of six. Nonetheless, this is standard fare at most daycare centers and is all too often what our children are given at home. Because these things are damp and hard to digest, they further impair the digestion and tend to cause phlegm and dampness which clog the system. When the flow of qi and blood which are inherently warm get blocked by phlegm and dampness, this heat is transferred to the pathologic accumulations thus causing damp heat and hot phlegm. Most food allergies manifest according to Chinese medicine as some version of heat and/or dampness and phlegm.

It is no wonder then that the foods which are most prone to causing food allergies are those which are the most dampening and phlegmatic. In a study conducted by Dr. Frederic Speer on 1,000 patients, he found that milk, chocolate, cola, corn, citrus, and egg were the most common food allergens. Milk allergies are especially common in children under two. Milk is very dampening according to Chinese dietary theory. Therefore, milk, cheese, and all dairy products tend to aggravate dampness and impede the spleen. If one's digestion is sound, these are very nutritious foods, but it is their very nutritiousness which also causes them to be dampening if one has insufficient spleen qi to distill their dampness.

Chocolate, which is extremely bitter, is rarely eaten alone. It is usually eaten in combination with sugar and tropical, hydrogenated oils. Chocolate by itself is warm and supplements the *ming men* or fire of life. When eaten with oils and sugars which are extremely dampening, chocolate tends to foster damp heat within the body. Again, this is especially the case with children whose digestion is not capable to transporting and transforming so much dampness and sweet.

Cola is made from a combination of sugars and spices, including cinnamon, citrus, and vanilla. These spices are warm and when eaten with foods are actually digestive aids. However, when taken with sugar water which overwhelms the baby's spleen, they too tend to cause damp heat.

Citrus fruits and juices are sweet and sour. These are the two flavors which in combination tend to be the most dampening according to Chinese five phase theory. Drinking the concentrated essence of oranges, grapefruit, pineapples, and lemons is like mainlining pathogenic dampness. This is especially the case in infants whose yang qi is still struggling to organize and permeate the dampness of their unstructured yin substance.

Corn is sweet with a neutral temperature according to Chinese medicine. It is this neutral temperature which makes corn difficult to digest in the newborn. Because corn lacks its own warmth and yet tends to be dampening because of its sweetness, and since the baby's spleen yang or warmth is weak, this dampness engendered by corn is difficult for the baby to transport and transform.

Eggs are likewise highly nutritious. They have a lot of *wei* as compared to qi. They are a wet, mucousy food which supplements yin and blood. This all adds up to a propensity to be dampening if one's fire of digestion does not burn strongly.

Other foods which cause food allergies and especially in children are soy products. Soybeans are sweet like corn but even cooler. They are quite dampening according to Chinese dietary theory. On the one hand, that makes them nutritious, but, on the other, that makes them hard to digest.

If one is fed or allowed to eat the wrong foods as a child, this can cause chronic spleen dampness and weakness. In Chinese medicine, it is said that dampness is heavy and turbid and hard to resolve. Once pathologic dampness is engendered in the spleen and body as a whole, it is difficult to rid. Therefore, dampness and phlegm engendered as a child may persist into adulthood, especially if one continues to eat the wrong, *i.e.*, damp and difficult to digest foods. When such foods are eaten, they cause even more dampness and possibly heat and the signs and symptoms of allergy appear.

Although Traditional Chinese Medicine has no category of disease called food allergies, its theory nonetheless explains why certain people experience certain signs and symptoms when they eat certain foods. Allergenic foods almost without exception tend to be dampening and hard to digest.

If one has such a food allergy, it is important to identify the worst offending foods and avoid these. At the same time, a warm, digestion-benefitting diet should be eaten to strengthen the spleen and transform and eliminate chronic dampness. It may take a seemingly long time, but eventually it is possible to strengthen the spleen and eliminate dampness to the point that a moderate amount of the previously allergenic foods can be added back into the diet. However, it should be noted that such highly nutritious, damp-tending foods should not be eaten too frequently nor in too large amounts by anyone. They are immoderate foods which tend to be too yin to eat too much of.

Candidiasis

Many Westerners suffer from candidiasis. Candidiasis is an overgrowth of intestinal yeast. *Candida albicans* are a normal, saprophytic yeast which live in the large intestine and act as scavengers metabolizing debris. However, if they proliferate out of control and if the lining of the intestines becomes too permeable, these yeast can infiltrate and migrate throughout the body. They can cause cystitis and vaginitis, sinusitis, thrush, skin diseases, and a host of other problems. Even if they just stay in the guts, they can cause chronic indigestion, flatulence, constipation or loose stools, fatigue, malaise, and depression.

In addition, overgrowth of *Candida albicans* can cause imbalance in the endocrine system. The endocrine system regulates the hormones and endocrine imbalance can disrupt the menstrual cycle in women causing PMS, early periods, and dysmenorrhea. The endocrine system also regulates the immune system and, therefore, candidiasis can play a very important role in chronic infectious diseases, various viral diseases, and in cancer.

Chinese medicine does recognize the existence of *Candida albicans*. TCM says that this parasite or *chong* in Chinese lives in the intestines and stomach. Further, Chinese medicine believes that it is excessive dampness and heat which provides the environment for run away proliferation of such *chong*. In TCM, candidiasis is always associated with spleen dampness and weakness with a tendency to damp heat. As we have seen above, dampness is caused by overeating foods which weaken the spleen and engender too much dampness. This includes sugar and refined carbohydrates and citrus fruits and juices. Damp heat *per se* is aggravated by alcohol which is both damp and hot.

Once one has candidiasis, it is important to stay away from eating any foods which tend to be spleen-weakening, damp-engendering, or damp heat-fostering. Also, one should avoid foods contaminated by yeast and fungus. This includes all fermented foods, all yeasted baked good, and anything with vinegar in it. Foods fermented with acidophilus, such as miso, are usually alright. However, because yogurt is made with milk and is, therefore, dampening, it may be contraindicated in certain individuals.

If one has a bad case of candidiasis, fungicidal medicines, whether these be herbal, pharmaceutical, or homeopathic, are often necessary as is bacterial replacement therapy with *Lactobacillus acidophilus* and *Bifidus bacterium*. Some authorities suggest a high protein diet but this may aggravate dampness and heat. Therefore, it is best to eat the basic healthy Chinese maintenance diet described in Chapter 2 but being careful to avoid all yeasted and fermented foods and all dampening, spleen-weakening foods. This means an emphasis on cooked vegetables and complex carbohydrates supplemented by some lean, animal protein.

There is more to say about the professional treatment of candidiasis. Interested readers are referred to my *Scatology & The Gate of Life: The Role of the Large Intestine in Immunity, An Integrated Chinese-Western Approach*. Other useful books

44

for the lay reader on candidiasis include William G. Crook's *The Yeast Connection* and Trowbridge & Walker's *The Yeast Syndrome*.

Cholesterol

H igh serum levels of cholesterol have become a national obsession in the United States. Many middle-aged and older Americans consciously attempt to eat a low cholesterol diet. However, the question of cholesterol includes some little understood facts. Although Traditional Chinese Medicine has no concept of cholesterol *per se*, still Western facts regarding cholesterol and diet can be seen through the lens of TCM.

Cholesterol is a nutrient in foods. It is a hormone precursor and so it is found especially in animal foods. Cholesterol is manufactured in our bodies as well as ingested when we eat. Its production is directly related to levels of stress. When we are under stress, our metabolism gears up. The orders for such gearing up are dependent upon hormonal regulation and many important hormones are synthesized from cholesterol. This is evidenced by the fact that many hormones have steroid or sterol in their name, such as the corticosteroids. This is the same sterol as in cholesterol.

The corticosteroids are manufactured in the adrenal cortex sitting on top of the kidneys. These corticosteroids are often referred to as flight or fight hormones. They are the hormones most closely associated with stress reactions in the body. Their manufacture is part of the body's coping mechanism for dealing with stresses of all kinds. What this means is that anything which stresses the body can cause an elevation in cholesterol production as a precursor to producing corticosteroids.

This means that high serum cholesterol levels are not simply a matter of high dietary cholesterol. A person's cholesterol is also a function of their level of stress. Eating sugar, drinking coffee and tea, and drinking alcohol are all stressful to the adrenal glands. From a Chinese medical point of view, coffee, tea, and alcohol liberate a lot of yang qi. Therefore, the body's response is to try to secrete more yin substance. Cholesterol is one such yin substance which becomes pathologic when excessive. Sugar, on the other hand, directly causes the secretion of yin damp-ness or pathologic substance.

Although eating a diet high in saturated fats can also cause the body to accumulate dampness and phlegm or pathologic yin substance, it is usually not necessary to become fanatical about avoiding all foods containing cholesterol. For instance, eggs have gotten a very bad rap lately because of their high choles-terol content. Chinese medicine believes that eggs are a very nutritious food. Specifically, they are a yin supplement. If a person is able to keep their level of stress under control and avoids sugar, alcohol, coffee, and tea, I believe they can eat a modicum of eggs and certainly more than many people think presently.

I have seen a number of patients with high cholesterol who were on very low cholesterol, restrictive diets and still could not get their cholesterol down. Within weeks after eliminating refined sugars and refined carbohydrates from their diets, all of these patients have been able to reduce their cholesterol levels to within safe limits. At that point, they were able to add back into their diet a modicum of cholesterol-containing foods, such as eggs, and their cholesterol did not increase as long as they avoided sugar.

Therefore, although I agree that one should not eat too many saturated fats, fatty meats, or too many eggs, avoiding sugar and sweets and reducing stress are equally important in maintaining healthy serum cholesterol levels. In TCM terms, cholesterol is a pure yin substance associated with the kidney *jing* or essence. However, when excessive, it becomes a pathologic yin composed of dampness and phlegm. Therefore, the key to keeping it under healthy control is to keep yang from becoming overly stressed and yin from being overly generated.

Obesity

I n Chinese medicine, fat is yin since it is an accumulation of substance. Specifically, TCM holds that fat or adipose tissue is mostly phlegm and dampness. As we have already seen, it is the Chinese spleen which is charged with transportation and transformation of dampness. It is also said in TCM that the spleen is the root of phlegm production. Therefore, Chinese dietary therapy's approach to the treatment of obesity revolves around improving the spleen's transportation and transformation of body fluids and its clean distillation of foods.

As mentioned previously, it is said in the *Nei Jing* that the *yang ming* begins to decline at around the age of 35. The *yang ming* means the stomach and intestines but also can stand for the entire process of digestion including Chinese spleen function. It is a well known fact that one's metabolism begins to slow down at around 40 and that, even if one eats the same foods and does the same exercise, it is not uncommon to put on 10 pounds or more at that time. The *Nei Jing* also says that in women at around 49 and in men at around 64, the kidneys begin their decline. The kidney fire or the *ming men zhi huo*, the fire of the gate of life, is the source of spleen yang or digestive fire. That means that a further gain in weight is also common as the kidneys produce less warmth and, therefore, the body's metabolism or warm transformations slow down even more.

The key to the Chinese dietary treatment of obesity, whether it be lifelong and congenital or due to aging, is to eat easily digestible foods and to keep the fire of digestion as strong and as efficient as possible. That means not eating too many sweet, damp, and greasy, fatty foods. It also means not eating cold foods or drinking cold liquids but rather drinking a small amount of warm liquids with meals. In addition, because the digestion becomes less efficient with age, it becomes all the more important not to overeat and, therefore, jam the qi mechanism.

Regular exercise keeps the qi, blood, and body fluids flowing. As the qi flows, the stomach and intestines conduct the dregs of foods and liquids downward for excretion. It is well known that exercise aids peristalsis and Chinese medical theory supports this fact. Exercise also warms the body up the same way that blowing on a dying fire can rekindle it. Regular, moderate exercise can significantly improve digestion and thus disinhibit the spleen's transportation or circulation of dampness and liquids and the spleen transformation of phlegm or fat. The word transform in Chinese is *hua*. *Hua* also means to melt. It implies a warm transformation. It is interesting to note that we also talk about melting fat away in colloquial English.

New diet programs come and go on a regular basis. Many of them just simply do not work for the majority of people. For instance, drinking copious amounts of cold water before meals in an attempt to fill oneself up only floods the spleen with more dampness. Likewise, drinking large amounts of grapefruit juice only causes the spleen to become damp, sodden, and inefficient. Some of the liquid diet programs currently available and highly touted can be good, but often they include psyllium seeds and oat bran which are both very dampening to the intestines according to Chinese dietary theory. When these are mixed with milk or citrus juices, they can be counterproductive regardless of the number of calories they provide. Although, outside the body, calories are calories, not all foods are digested the same way once inside the body. Professional practitioners of TCM can individually assess each patient's Chinese condition and should be able to tell if a particular diet plan or a particular meal replacement formula is appropriate for a given individual.

Even in Chinese medicine there are wise and less wise ways to go about shedding weight. Within Chinese herbal medicine, there are basically three approaches to weight loss. One approach is to give cold purgatives which essentially chill out the stomach/spleen so that food runs right through one. One loses weight because food is not digested after being eaten. However, since life is warm and since the stomach/spleen are the foundation of the latter heaven or postnatal acquisition of qi and blood, this is a risky approach. It can lead to chronic injury of the stomach/spleen in persons whose stomach/spleens are typically already functioning below par.

A second risky approach is to use pungent, warm, and dry diaphoretics which cause *jing* essence to be transformed into qi which is then dispersed upward and outward from the body. In this process, the lungs become hyperactive and discharge fluids and dampness through perspiration and urination. This method is essentially the Chinese equivalent of speed and can cause weakening of the kidneys, exhaustion of *jing* essence, and weakening of the lungs. If Olympic athletes use this method and these herbs, notably Herba Ephedrae (the vegetable source of ephedrine), they can be disqualified from their meets. This method is no different or safer than using dexedrin or methamphetamines.

The third approach which, in my opinion, is safer for more people is to use Chinese herbs which benefit digestion and gently seep dampness through increased urination but without causing either drastic purgation of the bowels or exhaustion of *jing* essence. Although the first two methods can be used safely by some patients for a limited length of time, they should be administered only on the basis of a professional TCM diagnosis and their use should be monitored continuously. Whereas, the third method of strengthening the spleen, disinhibiting dampness, and transforming phlegm can be safely employed by almost anyone.

It is believed in China that drinking moderate amounts of green tea with meals is very helpful to digestion and can reduce obesity. Green tea is unfermented, whereas black tea is cured and fermented. According to Chinese medicine, green tea strengthens the spleen and disinhibits dampness as well as transforms phlegm. Another helpful, dampness-disinhibiting tea can be made from Job's tears or coix, a Chinese barley. This grain, when taken as a dilute soup or decoction, also strengthens the spleen, disinhibits dampness, promotes drainage of pathologic dampness through urination, and seems to have some preventive ability against cancer.

Therefore, Chinese dietary therapy suggests that those struggling with unwanted weight should eat a diet high in lightly cooked vegetables, high in fiber and complex carbohydrates, mostly warm and easy to digest foods spiced with herbs that aid digestion, and should avoid foods which tend to be damp, phlegmatic, cold, or hard to digest. In addition, one should get more exercise and should consider getting acupuncture or Chinese herbal treatment to strengthen the fire of their digestion. Professional practitioners of Chinese medicine can also usually instruct patients in one or more systems of abdominal self-massage which can likewise stoke the fires of digestion and get the pot of the stomach boiling healthily again.

Coffee

I n Chinese medicine, coffee is classified as a bitter, pungent, and cold surface-relieving medicinal. Surface-relievers are basically diaphoretics. These medicinals work by transforming kidney yin or *jing* essence into qi which is then liberated up and outward through the system. As these move outward through the body's various energetic layers, they flood the organs within these layers with yang qi and so one experiences increased energy. In addition, this yang qi moving upward and outward promotes the flow of all the qi of the body, liberating stuck qi and with it activating blood and body fluids.

People who are either producing less qi from their daily diet, are using more qi through hyperactivity than they make each day, fail to store the qi they make because of disturbed sleep, or who lack access to their qi because of its being bound up or stagnant will all experience temporary access to abundant qi and the sense of energy and flow that go along with that when they drink coffee. However, because coffee is cool or cold energetically, it tends to chill the stomach/spleen or middle burner. This results in coffee's well known ability to move the stools and purge the intestines. Because coffee stimulates the lung's participation in the downward transportation of body fluids to the bladder, it is also a diuretic. Each time we urinate, we lose qi since urine does not just dribble out but is *yun*ned or transported. This means that we also lose warmth since qi is yang and, therefore, warm. Such purgation and diuresis weakens kidney yang at the same time as coffee steals kidney yin or *jing* essence.

Coffee, therefore, has a debilitating effect on both the middle and lower burners. Spleen yang is chilled and kidney yin and yang are exhausted. Using coffee as an energy boost is like continually dipping into one's savings or capital. Eventually such profligate deficit spending leaves one's internal economy bankrupt. When coffee transforms and liberates *jing* qi, one gets a rush but ultimately loses that precious stored energy.

When coffee was first introduced into Europe, there were prohibition movements and laws based on the recognition that coffee is a powerful and not wholly benign drug. Although coffee has certain legitimate medical and emergency uses, its use as a daily beverage is not very wise. It is my belief that if coffee were to be introduced to the West today as a new discovery, governmental agencies, such as the FDA in the United States, would restrict its use as a controlled substance. Since the government of the United States cannot, due to economic pressures, outlaw cigarette smoking which has incontestably been shown to be linked to lung cancer, it is even less likely that this common beverage could be prohibited at this late date. However, except as a medicinal and in cases where the use of speed is warranted knowing full well the risks its use entails, I believe coffee has no place in the diet of those hoping to be healthy. It is one of the few foods that I unequivocally deny to my patients.

Women especially do well to avoid coffee. Because of the violent upward dispersal coffee initiates in the body, it seems to injure the *chong mai*. The *chong mai* is an energy pathway running up the very core of the body connecting the kidneys to the heart. The purpose of this pathway is to feed kidney yang to the heart where it is transformed into the light of

58

consciousness or *shen ming*. It also leads kidney yin upwards to provide the nourishment and substantial support for the "higher" activities of consciousness and sensation. In injuring this connection between above and below, heart and kidneys, and exhausting yin, blood, and righteous body fluids, coffee tends to cause accumulations in women's breasts above and in their pelvises below. Although controlled tests do not confirm this fact, their results are, in my opinion, due to a flaw in their design and logic, since every astute clinician should know from experience that coffee negatively affects women's breasts and reproductive organs.

Vitamins

When I first began practicing TCM or Chinese medicine, I, like most converts to a new belief system, strove to hew to a very pure traditional Chinese practice. I perceived things like Western vitamin and mineral supplements as incompatible with such a pure, traditional approach. This was in the face of the fact that Chinese practitioners of TCM do not have any problem with using vitamin and mineral supplements. At that time, I confused Chinese medicine as a system of thought with medicines which come from China. These are not necessarily the same thing.

In Chinese medicine, probably as much as 20% of the standard repertoire of 500 medicinal substances originated outside of China. Spices such as cardamon, cloves, nutmeg, and cinnamon came from southeast and southwest Asia and the Spice Islands. Apricot, peach, and prune pits came from Central Asia and the Mideast. Licorice came from southern Russia. Sasparilla came from the Caribbean. Cinchona bark came from the Andes. Eagleswood, saffron, and terminalia came from India and the Himalayas. And American ginseng and greater celandine came from the United States and Canada.

In addition, Chinese medicinals, although referred to even in Chinese as *yao* or herbs, are not all herbal in origin. Rather they come from all three kingdoms -- animal, vegetable, and mineral. Further, Chinese doctors did not and do not only use naturally occurring medicinal substances found in their raw form. Chinese doctors and pharmacists have for centuries studied and employed a host of processing and refining techniques in order to make their medicinals more powerful and concentrated with less side effects and toxicity. So-called Chinese herbal medicine was largely the product of Daoist alchemists who were also the progenitors of the science of chemistry.

Therefore, there is no Chinese precedent for thinking that a practitioner of so-called Chinese medicine must only prescribe medicinals which originate in China, medicinals originating from vegetable or herbal sources, or naturally occurring substances in their raw or unprocessed form. That means there is no *a priori* reason vitamins and minerals cannot be incorporated into the contemporary practice of Traditional Chinese Medicine.

When vitamins, minerals, amino acids, enzymes, co-enzymes, fatty acids, and co-factors are used medicinally, these are referred to as orthomolecular supplements. Orthomolecular means the same molecules as the body itself. Orthomolecular supplements are essentially concentrations of nutrient substances normally found in the foods we eat. Many people ask, if this is so, if vitamins and minerals are simply found in the foods we eat, why can't we get enough of these in our daily diet? That is a good question but one which can be easily answered.

First of all, many people in the West do not eat a healthy and balanced diet. We tend not to eat enough fresh vegetables and we tend to eat too much sugar, protein, and fats. These foods cause us to use up inordinate amounts of certain other nutrients. For instance, if one eats lots of meat, one needs more calcium. And sugar causes us to use up more zinc.

Secondly, many of the foods we eat are grown in poor soil due to excessive use of chemical fertilizers and other modern but short-sighted farming practices. This is compounded by the fact that many people today eat foods which have been prepared and stored by canning, freezing, and dehydrating which cause some loss of vitamins and enzymes.

Third, we are exposed to toxic chemicals in our air, water, and food which are a type of extra stress on our systems requiring extra nutrients to neutralize these.

Fourth, most of us living in urban environments are subject to large amounts of mental and emotional stress. It is my belief that simply living in the urban West is more than our nervous systems are capable of dealing with in a healthy way. There are just too many and unrelieved stresses which are constantly assaulting us. Such stress uses up inordinate amounts of B vitamins and minerals.

Fifth, if one drinks coffee or alcohol, smokes cigarettes, is exposed to radiation, is taking certain medications, such as oral birth control pills, or is suffering from a chronic illness, and especially a digestive complaint, either one is using up abnormally large amounts of certain nutrients or is not absorbing others from their food.

For all these reasons, one may need to supplement certain nutrients which are not adequately found in their diet. This does not mean that if one gobbles lots of vitamins one does not need to eat a healthy diet. What it does mean is that, given the stressful, polluted world we live in, we may not be getting enough vital nutrients simply from our diet.

In the last couple of years I have worked out the TCM descriptions of all the common vitamins, minerals, and amino acids. These have been published in my *Something Old, Something New: Essays on the TCM Description of Western Herbs, Pharmaceuticals, Vitamins & Minerals*. Using these descriptions, Western practitioners of TCM can prescribe orthomolecular supplements based on a TCM diagnosis just as if they were prescribing Chinese herbs. Although this is not something I suggest laypersons do for themselves, I have included this brief discussion of orthomolecular supplements in this layperson's guide to Chinese dietary therapy primarily to let patients know that such supplements are consistent with the practice of TCM. They are a useful adjunct to other, more standard TCM therapies and should not be overlooked simply because they are not "Chinese". This is a definite evolution from my position on vitamins and minerals when I wrote *Prince Wen Hui's Cook* in 1982.

Conclusion

While preparing this small book on Chinese dietary therapy for laypersons, I have coincidentally come across two things that support and underscore the importance of this approach. The first is a scientific study comparing the eating habits of 6,500 rural Chinese and their health with Western eating habits and our health. This study was undertaken jointly by Oxford University, the Chinese Academy for Preventive Medicine in Beijing, and Cornell University. This is the largest study of a nation's eating habits of this kind ever undertaken.

For two years, the subjects, aged between 34-64, were interviewed about their eating and other health habits, such as drinking and smoking. Blood samples were taken to measure cholesterol and other such things, dietary records were obtained, and foods consumed were weighed and measured. Among the important finding were the facts that:

1. The Chinese consume many more vegetables, grains, and fruits than Americans or Britons.

2. The daily fiber intake of the average Chinese is 3 times that of the average American.

3. The average Chinese derives anywhere from 6-24% of their

daily calories from fat, compared to 39% for the average American and 45% for the average Briton.

4. In most of the counties included in this study, people eat meat only about once a week. In counties where meat is eaten regularly, rates of cardiovascular disease are also higher.

5. The Chinese eat more calories daily than Americans per pound of body weight but suffer little obesity.

6. The average Chinese blood cholesterol level is only 127 milligrams per deciliter compared to 212 in the United States.

90% of the Chinese selected for this study were provincials who ate locally raised foods and stuck to a traditional diet. I believe this study supports the fact that the Chinese do have a special insight into diet and the maintenance of health. Based on the outcome of this study, the Chinese government is currently taking active steps to keep this traditional diet from giving way to the high-fat diet of the West.

The second piece of interesting evidence supporting the wisdom of the Chinese medical approach to healthy eating was recently published in *Newsweek* (May 27, 1991). The cover article of this issue was devoted to new attitudes about diet and health in the United States. According to that article, the USDA has created what it calls "The Eating Right Pyramid". This is a graphic showing, in its preparers opinion, the most healthy proportions of foods in one's daily diet. This pyramid makes grains and complex carbohydrates the foundation of the diet. Next comes vegetables and fruits. Then comes dairy products and other animal proteins, and last, under the heading "Use Sparingly" comes fats, oils, and sweets.

This is very similar to the diet that Chinese medicine suggests is the healthiest for humans living in temperate climates. The only change I would make in this scheme is that I would emphasize more vegetables, since, as a clinician, I know that even those Westerners trying to eat a healthy diet tend to eat

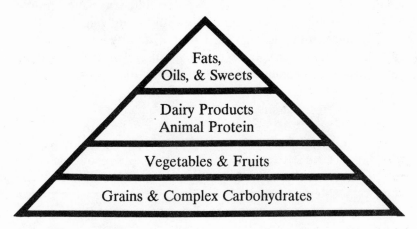

too many grain products and too few vegetables. The same article quotes Bonnie Liebman, a nutritionist at the Center for Science in the Public Interest, as saying: "For years, the National Academy of Sciences and the National Cancer Institute have been telling Americans to eat more vegetables." Says CSPI's Liebman, "Most of the meal should be grains, vegetables and beans, and meats should be used as a condiment." Unfortunately but all too typically, Secretary of Agriculture, Edward R. Madigan, suspended the publication of this chart presumably due to special interest pressure from the meat and dairy industries.

For sure, some "truths" are culturally limited. Certain mores and behavior may work in one culture or country but not in others. However, Chinese medicine is a system of thought about human physiology which is so universally valid that its logic can be applied to any person within any culture in the world. Chinese internal medicine is not simply a collection of medicinals which happen to have originated in China, nor is Chinese dietary therapy limited to wontons and egg drop soup. The fundamental insights of Chinese dietary theory can be applied to any national or regional cuisine since all foods in everyone's stomachs must be turned into 100° soup.

Although more and more, Western science supports the diet rural Chinese have been eating for millennia, the facts of Western science are not something immediately experiencable on a human level. Cholesterol, enzymes, proteins, etc. are so removed from everyday experience that people are prone to unconsciously dismiss them even if, theoretically, they know about them. For most people, these facts exist only as vague abstractions. Chinese medicine, on the other hand, has crafted its theories from metaphors taken from everyday reality. This is based on the perception that whatever goes on within the body is not something apart or different from what goes on in the world at large.

Chinese medicine is based on the concept that the human organism is a microcosm of the larger, external macrocosm. As a holographic part of this macrocosm, one can apply the same everyday metaphors one uses to understand the world at large to their own insides. Therefore, the analogies between digestion and a pot on a stove, to a car engine, a still, and to Economics 101 are both accurate and empowering if seemingly simplistic. My experience as a clinician is that such explanations are able to influence the behavior of patients that more abstract explanations often cannot. It is my experience that when we really apprehend something as being immediately and undeniably true, we tend to act upon that belief.

Chinese dietary therapy gives us a set of explanations from our normal, everyday world. These explanations make sense and, more than that, when they are put into action, they work. As a human being and a doctor, there are many things which I say I believe but really do not know for sure. But, when it comes to diet, I do know for sure that the wisdom of Chinese dietary therapy does work. I also know that diet is such an important part of our daily life and existence that unless one's diet is well adjusted and appropriately regulated, no amount of herbs, acupuncture, or other medicines or treatments can achieve a complete and lasting cure. Therefore, whether for prevention or remedial treatment, proper diet is of utmost importance, and dietary wisdom is something that everyone needs to know. Chinese medicine has that wisdom. Good luck.

Bibliography

Flaws, Bob, *Food, Phlegm, & Pediatric Disease*, Blue Poppy Press, Boulder, CO, 1990

Flaws, Bob & Wolfe, Honora Lee, *Prince Wen Hui's Cook: Chinese Dietary Therapy*, Paradigm Publications, Brookline, MA 1983

Flaws, Bob, *Scatology & The Gate of Life: The Role of the Large Intestine in Immunity, An Integrated Chinese-Western Approach*, Blue Popp Press, Boulder, CO, 1990

Flaws, Bob, *Something Old, Something New: Essays on the TCM Description of Western Herbs, Pharmaceuticals, Vitamins & Minerals*, Blue Poppy Press, Boulder, CO 1991

Kaptchuk, Ted, *The Web That Has No Weaver*, Congden & Weed, New York, 1984

Korngold, Efrem & Beinfeld, Harriet, *Between Heaven and Earth*, Ballantine, New York, 1991

OTHER BOOKS ON CHINESE MEDICINE AVAILABLE FROM BLUE POPPY PRESS

1775 Linden Ave
Boulder, CO 80304
PH. 303\442-0796 FAX 303\447-0740

PMS: Its Cause, Diagnosis & Treatment According to Traditional Chinese Medicine by Bob Flaws ISBN 0-936185-22-8 $14.95

SOMETHING OLD, SOMETHING NEW; Essays on the TCM Description of Western Herbs, Pharmaceuticals, Vitamins & Minerals by Bob Flaws ISBN 0-936185-21-X $19.95

SCATOLOGY & THE GATE OF LIFE: The Role of the Large Intestine in Immunity, An Integrated Chinese-Western Approach by Bob Flaws ISBN 0-936185-20-1 $12.95

SECOND SPRING: A Guide To Healthy Menopause Through Traditional Chinese Medicine by Honora Lee Wolfe ISBN 0-936185-18-X $14.95

MIGRAINES & TRADITIONAL CHINESE MEDICINE: A Layperson's Guide by Bob Flaws ISBN 0-936185-15-5 $11.95

STICKING TO THE POINT: A Rational Methodology for the Step by Step Formulation & Administration of an Acupuncture Treatment by Bob Flaws ISBN 0-936185-17-1 $14.95

ENDOMETRIOSIS & INFERTILITY AND TRADITIONAL CHINESE MEDICINE: A Laywoman's Guide by Bob Flaws ISBN 0-936185-14-7 $9.95

CLASSICAL MOXIBUSTION SKILLS IN CONTEMPORARY CLINICAL PRACTICE by Sung Baek ISBN 0-936185-16-3 $10.95

THE BREAST CONNECTION: A Laywoman's Guide to the Treatment of Breast Disease by Chinese Medicine by Honora Lee Wolfe ISBN 0-936185-13-9 $8.95

NINE OUNCES: A Nine Part Program For The Prevention of AIDS in HIV Positive Persons by Bob Flaws ISBN 0-936185-12-0 $9.95

THE TREATMENT OF CANCER BY INTEGRATED CHINESE-WESTERN MEDICINE by Zhang Dai-zhao, trans. by Zhang Ting-liang & Bob Flaws, ISBN 0-936185-11-2 $16.95

BLUE POPPY ESSAYS: 1988 Translations and Ruminations on Chinese Medicine by Flaws, Chace et al, ISBN 0-936185-10-4 $18.95

A HANDBOOK OF TRADITIONAL CHINESE DERMATOLOGY by Liang Jian-hui, trans. by Zhang Ting-liang & Bob Flaws, ISBN 0-936185-07-4 $14.95

SECRET SHAOLIN FORMULAE FOR THE TREATMENT OF EXTERNAL INJURY by Patriarch De Chan, trans. by Zhang Ting-liang & Bob Flaws, ISBN 0-936185-08-2 $13.95

A HANDBOOK OF TRADITIONAL CHINESE GYNECOLOGY by Zhejiang College of TCM, trans. by Zhang Ting-liang, ISBN 0-936185-06-6 (2nd edit.) $21.95

FREE & EASY: Traditional Chinese Gynecology for American Women 2nd Edition, by Bob Flaws, ISBN 0-936185-05-8 $15.95

PRINCE WEN HUI'S COOK: Chinese Dietary Therapy by Bob Flaws & Honora Lee Wolfe, ISBN 0-912111-05-4, $12.95 (Published by Paradigm Press, Brookline, MA)

TURTLE TAIL & OTHER TENDER MERCIES: Traditional Chinese Pediatrics by Bob Flaws ISBN 0-936185-00-7 $14.95

THE DAO OF INCREASING LONGEVITY AND CONSERVING ONE'S LIFE by Anna Lin & Bob Flaws, ISBN 0-936185-24-4 $16.95

FIRE IN THE VALLEY: The TCM Diagnosis and Treatment of Vaginal Diseases by Bob Flaws ISBN 0-936185-25-2 $16.95

HIGHLIGHTS OF ANCIENT ACUPUNCTURE PRESCRIPTIONS trans. by Honora Lee Wolfe & Rose Crescenz ISBN 0-936185-23-6 $14.95

About the Author

Bob Flaws, DOM, CMT, Dipl.Ac. is author or translator of over two dozen books on Chinese medicine. In addition, Dr. Flaws is an internationally known practitioner of Traditional Chinese Medicine specializing in gynecological complaints. He has studied acupuncture, *tuina* (Chinese remedial massage), and Chinese herbal medicine at the Shanghai College of TCM and is also a graduate of the Boulder School of Massage Therapy. Among his many other credits are the founding of Blue Poppy Press, a publishing company devoted to the printing and distribution of books on all aspects of Oriental medicine. Dr. Flaws regularly lectures at schools and conferences in the US, UK, Australia, and New Zealand.